W9-BPM-905

Clerical and Data Management for the Pharmacy Technician

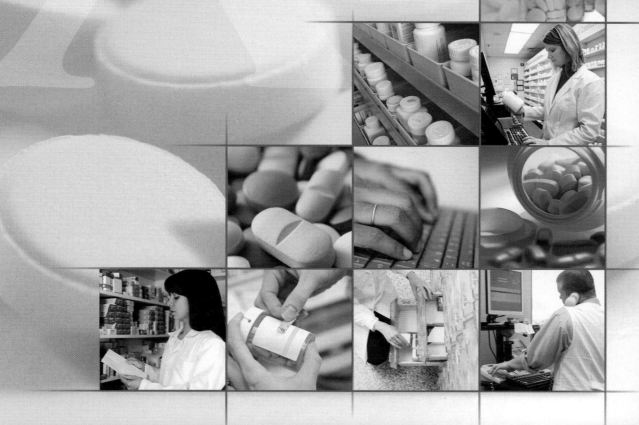

Clerical and Data Management for the Pharmacy Technician

Linda Quiett

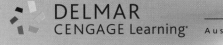

DELMAR
CENGAGE Learning·   Australia Canada Mexico Singapore Spain United Kingdom United States

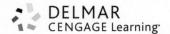
DELMAR
CENGAGE Learning·

Clerical and Data Management for the Pharmacy Technician
Linda Quiett

Vice President, Editorial: Dave Garza

Director of Learning Solutions: Matthew Kane

Acquisitions Editor: Tari Broderick

Managing Editor: Marah Bellegarde

Senior Product Manager: Darcy M. Scelsi

Editorial Assistant: Nicole Manikas

Vice President, Marketing: Jennifer Baker

Marketing Manager: Jonathan Sheehan

Senior Director, Education Production:
Wendy A. Troeger

Production Manager: Andrew Crouth

Senior Content Project Manager: Kara A. DiCaterino

Senior Art Director: Jack Pendleton

Technology Project Manager: Jim Gilbert

© 2012 Delmar, Cengage Learning

ALL RIGHTS RESERVED. No part of this work covered by the copyright herein may be reproduced, transmitted, stored, or used in any form or by any means graphic, electronic, or mechanical, including but not limited to photocopying, recording, scanning, digitizing, taping, Web distribution, information networks, or information storage and retrieval systems, except as permitted under Section 107 or 108 of the 1976 United States Copyright Act, without the prior written permission of the publisher.

For product information and technology assistance, contact us at
Cengage Learning Customer & Sales Support, 1-800-354-9706

For permission to use material from this text or product,
submit all requests online at **www.cengage.com/permissions.**
Further permissions questions can be e-mailed to
permissionrequest@cengage.com

ApotheSoft-Rx ® is a registered trademark of the ApotheSoft, LLC.

Library of Congress Control Number: 2011942791

ISBN-13: 978-1-4390-5781-0

ISBN-10: 1-4390-5781-8

Delmar
5 Maxwell Drive
Clifton Park, NY 12065-2919
USA

Cengage Learning is a leading provider of customized learning solutions with office locations around the globe, including Singapore, the United Kingdom, Australia, Mexico, Brazil, and Japan. Locate your local office at:
international.cengage.com/region

Cengage Learning products are represented in Canada by Nelson Education, Ltd..

To learn more about Delmar, visit **www.cengage.com/delmar**

Purchase any of our products at your local college store or at our preferred online store **www.cengagebrain.com**

Notice to the Reader

Publisher does not warrant or guarantee any of the products described herein or perform any independent analysis in connection with any of the product information contained herein. Publisher does not assume, and expressly disclaims, any obligation to obtain and include information other than that provided to it by the manufacturer. The reader is expressly warned to consider and adopt all safety precautions that might be indicated by the activities described herein and to avoid all potential hazards. By following the instructions contained herein, the reader willingly assumes all risks in connection with such instructions. The publisher makes no representations or warranties of any kind, including but not limited to, the warranties of fitness for particular purpose or merchantability, nor are any such representations implied with respect to the material set forth herein, and the publisher takes no responsibility with respect to such material. The publisher shall not be liable for any special, consequential, or exemplary damages resulting, in whole or part, from the readers' use of, or reliance upon, this material.

Printed in China
2 3 4 5 6 7 17 16 15 14

Dedication

My first job as a pharmacy technician was with a long-term care pharmacy that was establishing a new branch in Florida. At that time, I had good basic skills, but I knew absolutely nothing about handling patient data. Fortunately, I had the distinct pleasure to work with one of the greatest pharmacists I have ever had an opportunity to know. When James Jawor, RPh, came to the pharmacy, everyone's life changed. He spent time with each of the pharmacy technicians, explaining how things were to be done correctly. The qualities that made him exceptional were his patience and his willingness to correct a mistake and explain why it was a mistake and how to correct it.

When working with James, there was also never a dull moment. If he was checking labels before they went out on the floor for packing or checking the final product before it was to be delivered to the nursing homes, he always offered a good joke and a history lesson about pharmacy work. I will always remember his polite way of correcting an error on an order entry. He would start out with, "Now, Missy" and then proceed to explain what was wrong with the entry.

We still communicate to this day. James has retired to spend more time with his lovely wife, children, and grandchildren. For all he did to improve my work experience and learning, I dedicate this book to Jim.

TABLE OF CONTENTS

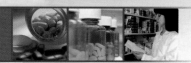

PREFACE

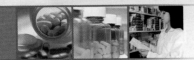

Clerical and Data Management for the Pharmacy Technician was conceived to fill the gap for pharmacy technicians who are in school and need further instruction to make a successful transition to the work environment. Fortunately, all of the many different work environments require basic knowledge about data management.

In today's computerized world of information, it may be easy to assume that the computer will handle everything for us. Well, computerization does help with the massive workload in pharmaceutical care, but the operator—pharmacist, pharmacy technician, physician, or nurse—has to enter the information into the computer. The computer then takes that information and completes several functions simultaneously to save time. But the information being entered into the computer has to be correct. The intent of this text is to help you understand that process, how the computer takes the information and manipulates it into usable formats.

The ApotheSoft-Rx© software was written by a retail pharmacist and is in use in many pharmacies. Throughout their careers, pharmacy technicians will be exposed to different software in different settings, some proprietary and others from different providers. Whatever the case, the basics are the same as presented here.

The chapters in this book offer hands-on practice in entering new patient information, physicians information, inputting inventory, entering insurance claims, and entering compounds. The aim is to provide an overview of what is to be expected when handling patient information, emphasizing the importance of attention to detail.

This book may be used by the beginning pharmacy student, pharmacy technician, or store manager. It is accompanied by a CD that will allow for building patient files, doctor information, inventory, and compounds. The program is applicable to retail, long-term care, and hospital pharmacies.

ABOUT THE AUTHOR

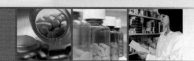

Linda Quiett, BA, CPhT, has more than 15 years of experience in long-term care pharmacy practice. She also has taught in associate degree and certificate pharmacy technology programs. Ms. Quiett holds a Bachelor of Arts degree in education from the University of South Florida, an Associate of Science degree in Medical Laboratory Technology from St. Petersburg College, Florida, and a Certificate in Pharmacy Technology from the Pinellas Technical Education Centers, Florida. She is a member of several national pharmacy and pharmacy technician organizations:

Pharmacy Technician Educators Council

Amerian Society of Health-System Pharmacists

American Pharmacists Association

National Pharmacy Technician Association

American Association of Pharmacy Technicians

ACKNOWLEDGEMENTS

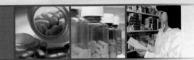

Thank you to all of the pharmacy technicians and pharmacists I have had the pleasure of working with and training over the years while working in pharmacy and teaching. Your work will be a continuous learning experience for you, and may you continue to increase your knowledge in the future.

A special thank you to Gayle Holbrook, B.A., CPhT, whose encouragement kept me going. An extra special thank you to Marty Francom for his development of the software program and assistance to me before and during the writing of this book.

REVIEWERS

Melinda Alam, CPhT
Charter College—Canyon Country
Canyon Country, California

Joseph P. Gee, PharmD, RPh
Consumnes River College
Sacramento, California

Brooke Irving Haver, CPhT
Jefferson Union High School
Daly City, California

INTRODUCTION

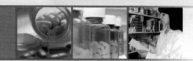

As a pharmacy technician, you will be called upon to perform many tasks to assist the pharmacist in pharmacy operations. Among the most essential of these roles are data management and use of the pharmacy software system.

Various pharmacy software operating systems are used throughout the many practice settings of pharmacy. The software program you will use in this book is ApotheSoft-Rx, a functioning program written and developed by a pharmacist and is in widespread use.

The aim of this book is to familiarize pharmacy technicians with the basics of data management and requirements in the day-to-day operation of the pharmacy. Pharmacy technicians may be exposed to several different software operating systems and may have to learn a new system if the pharmacy changes software vendors or upgrades the current system, or if they change work locations. Still, every system is basically the same, and the information is simply entered in a different manner through different screens. With the basic information presented here, such a transition should not be difficult.

Before starting to work through each chapter, the ApotheSoft-Rx program must be opened on your computer. The program may have been installed on your school computer already, and your instructor may give you instructions before you open the program. If this program is not already loaded, do so now.

INSTALLING THE PROGRAM

A CD-ROM accompanies this text and can be found on the inside back cover. Insert the CD into the CD-ROM drive. In most instances, the program will begin to install automatically. If the program does not start automatically, click on **Start**, and then click **Run**. The **Run** dialog box will open. In the **Open** text box, type d:\demosetup.exe (where **d** is the drive letter of your CD or DVD drive).

After the program begins to install, the following screen will appear (Figure I-1). Be sure to read the information in each screen carefully, and then click **Next** and proceed to the next screen.

The **License Agreement** (Figure I-2) will appear. Although you may or may not see this agreement on the software you will be using at your pharmacy, you should understand that in most cases the software is being leased from the software provider. Any misuse of the software could endanger the pharmacy financially; the software company would be able to bring a lawsuit against the pharmacy and demand a large financial settlement for misuse of its software product.

You will notice that "I do not accept the agreement" is checked. After reading the agreement, check "I accept the agreement" and click the **Next** button to move to the next screen.

An **Information** screen (Figure I-3) will open. Read the information about the program, then click on **Next**.

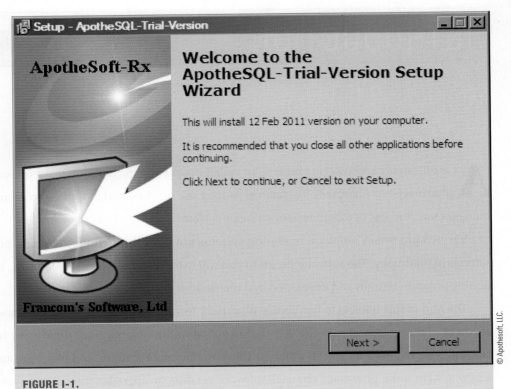

FIGURE I-1.

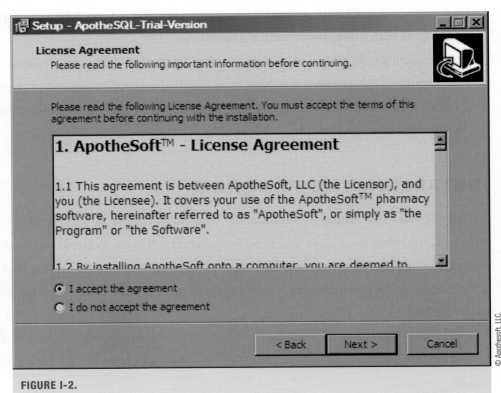

FIGURE I-2.

The **Ready to In-stall** (Figure I-4) screen will appear. Click on the **Install** button, and the installation will start.

The **Installing** screen (Figure I-5) will appear, and the bars will proceed across as the files are loaded onto your computer.

After the installation is complete, a small box will appear, pertaining to the **License Download**. Click **OK** and another box, **Success**, will appear.

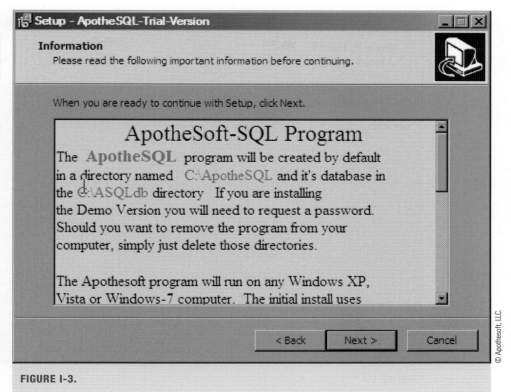

FIGURE I-3.

© Apothesoft, LLC.

Click **OK**, and another box, **Licenses & Expirations**, will appear (Figure I-6A, 6B, and 6C). These three boxes pertain to the pharmacy's licensing agreement with the ApotheSoft provider.

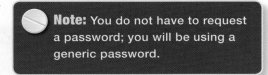

Note: You do not have to request a password; you will be using a generic password.

In the **Licenses & Expirations** box, notice a license for Offsite Backup storage and Lexi (referring to Lexicomp—a company that, by subscription, provides information to healthcare professionals to aid them in making safer and faster decisions with easy-to-use clinical information (e.g., drug interactions, diet information, and colored pictures of each drug product). Offsite Backup storage refers to backing up the pharmacy files at the end of each day. When you shut down the program, a box appears asking if you want to back up the files. You should always answer no because there is no license agreement with ApotheSoft to back up your files.

After you have OK'd all three boxes, another **Information** screen (Figure I-7) will appear. Read the information in the box, but remember—you do not have to request a password. If your instructor does not provide you with a password, use the default. The default password is **rph** all in lowercase letters.

After you have read the Information and clicked the **Next** button, the final setup screen will appear (Figure I-8). After reading the screen, click on the **Finish** button. The screen states that you may select the installed icon to launch the program.

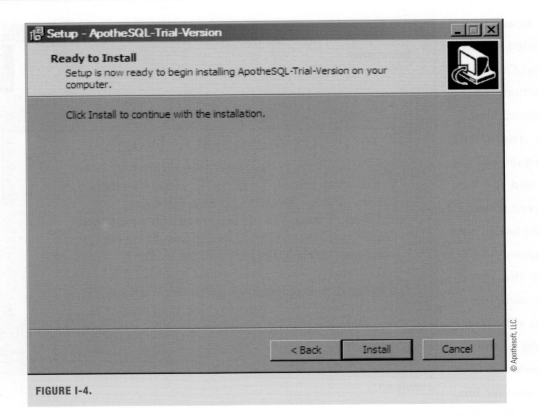

FIGURE I-4.

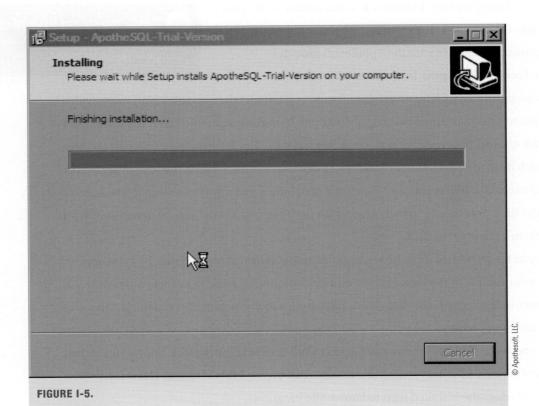

FIGURE I-5.

If the icon does not appear on your desktop, you may access it by going to the **Start** menu and clicking on Programs. In the programs list, select the ApotheSoft program. From the drop-down list, select ApotheSoft, and the program will launch. If the program does not appear on the desktop, it might also appear in your **Start** menu,.

After you open the program, a screen with ApotheSoft-Rx will appear at the top (Figure I-9). This is the sign-in screen. You may want to scroll through all of the screens by clicking on the **Next** button and reviewing the material. Some of the information pertains to functions to which you may or may not have access. After reviewing the screens, enter the information requested in the **Set RPH** box, which will allow for you to enter the pharmacist's initials

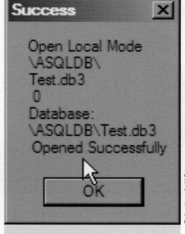

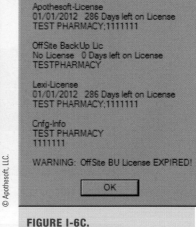

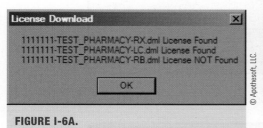

FIGURE I-6A.

FIGURE I-6B.

FIGURE I-6C.

FIGURE I-7.

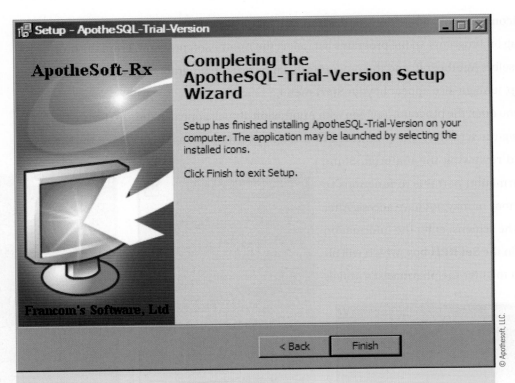

© Apothesoft, LLC.

FIGURE I-8.

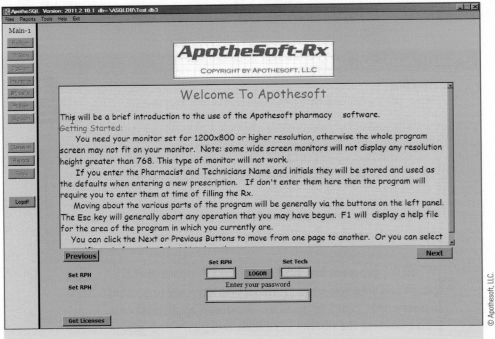

© Apothesoft, LLC.

FIGURE I-9.

or name, and in the **Set Tech** box, which will allow you to enter your initials or name.

Remember: The password is **rph**, all lowercase.

After you have reviewed the different screens, set **RPH** and **Tech** and enter the password (Figure I-10), which is all lowercase, then press ENTER.

The first screen to appear (Figure I-11) will be the Prescription screen, which will allow you to refill or fill prescriptions. This, however, is only one of the screens you will use to manage patient data in the pharmacy's day-to-day operation.

In short, as a pharmacy technician, you may use many different computer software programs, but the information data to be managed are always the same or similar.

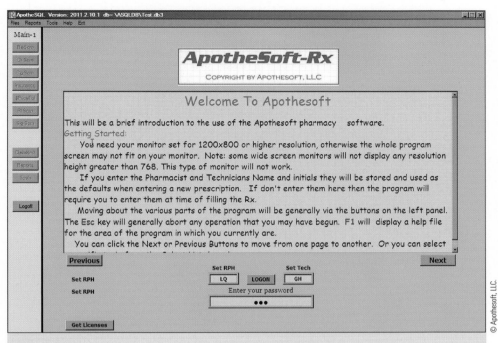

FIGURE I-10.

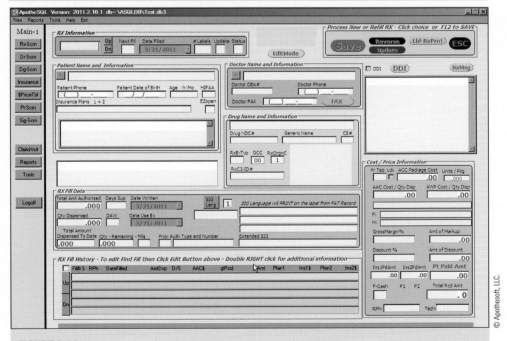

FIGURE I-11.

> **Note:** Whenever you are not using the computer, it is good practice to log off. This will prevent another pharmacist or pharmacy technician from entering data in your working screen.

CHAPTER 1

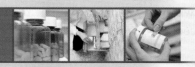

Entering a New Patient

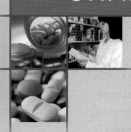

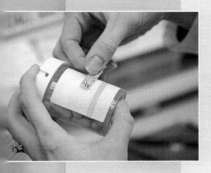

LEARNING OBJECTIVES

Describe the procedures to follow when receiving a new patient medication order or prescription.

1. Explain the importance of the patient miscellaneous information.

2. Discuss the importance of entering patient allergies and medical conditions.

3. Explain when and why a patient's information may be edited.

4. Discuss why ICD-9 codes are used to indicate allergies and medical conditions.

Entering patient information into the pharmacy computer correctly is vital to efficient operation of the pharmacy. Without this information, the patient may be at risk for incurring a drug-related adverse reaction, not receiving the correct medication, or being billed improperly for medications and medical supplies. Many other errors are possible, too, which explains the necessity of entering all new patient information and editing existing patients correctly. This chapter addresses some of the processes involved in entering new patient information, including the patient's allergies and medical conditions.

When first entering a new patient into the database, the pharmacy technician logs on to the ApotheSoft-Rx program. The instructor may have provided the initials and password for you to use. If not, use the pharmacist's initials, the pharmacy technician's initials, and create a password. After you are logged on, familiarize yourself with the software's various screens in **Main-1** (Figure 1-1). Move from the **Rx-Scrn** button to the **Pt-Scrn** button by clicking on the buttons on the left side of the

Main-1

Rx-Scrn

Dr-Scrn

Dg-Scrn

Insurance

$PriceTbl

Pt-Scrn

Sig-Scrn

ClaimXmit

Reports

Tools

Logoff

© Apothesoft, LLC.

FIGURE 1-1.

screen. The button **ClaimXmit** will take you out of **Main-1**. You will work with each of the screens shown in Figure 1-1 as you proceed through the chapters.

PHYSICIAN'S ORDER

After you have acquainted yourself briefly with each of the screens, look at the Physician's Order form (Figure 1-2). This is a typical example of an order that would be received by fax by a pharmacy supplying medication to a long-term care Skilled Nursing Facility. As a pharmacy technician, you will see various types of forms used to request medications for a patient. Examples of different types of patient profiles or orders are given in Appendix A.

Begin by looking over the patient information in Figure 1-2. *A requisite for pharmacy technicians is to ensure that the information is as correct and complete as possible.* This is an example of the orders for a patient residing in Waterford SNF, a Skilled Nursing Facility for patients requiring care over a long period of time. Note the location of the resident name, room number, date of birth, Social Security number, physician, and the physician's phone number. Upon receipt of this form, the pharmacy technician immediately checks to make sure that it is complete. If it is not, the technician is to call the nursing facility to obtain the missing information. An example of complete information is as follows.

```
Resident Name: Sallie Mae Jones
Rm#: 114D
Date of Birth: 7/15/1925
SSN#: 266-89-3333
Dr: Scott Smith, M.D.
Phone: 423-555-0135
```

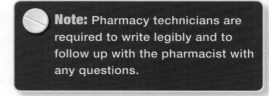

Note: Pharmacy technicians are required to write legibly and to follow up with the pharmacist with any questions.

ENTERING PATIENT INFORMATION

Starting from the **Main-1** menu buttons on the left side of the screen, navigate to the **Pt-Scrn** button and click with the mouse on that button. This will bring up the **Patient Identification Information** screen (Figure 1-3).

Look at the information requested on the screen, the information available on the Physician's Order form, and the information you received when you called the nursing facility. The one piece of information you did not receive was the PAYTYPE, which is checked Medicare on the form. This information will be handled at a later date.

Next search for the patient to be sure that the patient is not in the system already. To do this, begin typing the first few letters of the patient's last name in the **Patient Search** box inside the **Patient Identification Information** box. If a patient with the same last name comes up in the **Patient Name Search List**, check the date of birth, sex, and any other information available to be sure this is the correct patient and thereby avoid an error. Individuals with the same name are common, so care is necessary. If the patient is not already in the system, add the patient.

DATE
01/16/XX

Resident PRN, ORDERS
Name:

PHYSICIAN'S ORDER

ORIGINAL

ORDERS	FREQ.

OTHER ODERS

D/C _____ Order# 00002
01) TYLENOL 5GR TABLET — GIVE 2 TABLETS (10CC)
PO EVERY 4 HOURS AS NEEDED FOR PAIN/TEMP >101
(OR SUPP)
ICD9 Diagnosis **0.9 GENERAL SYMPTOMS REC**

D/C _____ Order# 00001
02) MILK OF MEGNESIA — GIVE 30ML PO EVERY 3 DAYS
AS NEEDED IF NO IM
ICD9 Diagnosis **4.0 CONSTIPATION**

D/C _____ Order# 00004
03) DULCULAR SUPPOSITORY — INSERT 1 SUPP.
RECTALLY EVERY 4TH DAY AS NEEDED IF NO B.M.
ICD9 Diagnosis **4.0 CONSTIPATION**

XANAX 0.25mg PO XXXX HS — 9P
ICD9 Diagnosis **ANXIETY**

DIGOXIN 0.25mg PO QY — 9A
ICD9 Diagnosis **TACHYCORDIC**

CARDIZEM CD 120mg PO QY — 9A
ICD9 Diagnosis **HEAT DYALYSIS**

AGGREWOX, PO B XXXX — 9B / 9P
ICD9 Diagnosis

XXXXXX 100mg PO, CAP B XXXX — 9A / SP
ICD9 Diagnosis

DIAGNOSIS   XXXXXXXXXXXX XXXXXXXXXXX XXXXX XXXXXXX XXXXX
XXXXXXXXXXXXX XXXX

DOCTOR   DATE   6/25/XX
                ROOM #   112/D
RESIDENT   ALLERGIES XXXXXXXXXXX
                           XXXXXXXXXXX
                           XXXXXX

XXXX REVISION DATE: 01-27-20XX
ADMIT TO WATERFORD SNF DATE:_____
RESIDENT NAME:_____
RM.#_____
DATE OF BIRTH:_____
SSN#:_____
DR:_____
PHONE:_____
PAYTYPE:
(✓)-MEDICARE (XXXXXX)
(_)-MEDICAID/MEDICAID PEND (XXXX)
(_)-MANAGED CARE - SKILLED (MGD)
(_)-PRIVATE (PVTEX)
(_)-IMSPICE:_____
(_)-VA (VA)
(_)-INSURANCE/AMC - NON-SKILLED
_____

DIET ORDERS:
DIET: NCS _____

FOOD/BEVERAGE EXCEPTIONS:
(✓)-YES   (_)-NO........ DIETARY LIBERTY FOR
SPECIAL OCCASIONS (S-CPDIETLIB)

(_)-YES   (X)-NO........ ALCOHOLIC BEVERAGES AT
SPECIAL OCCASIONS (S-CPETON)

ANCILLARY ORDERS:
(✓)-SKILLED. (_)-INTERMEDIATE... LEVEL OF CASE
(_)-GOOD. (_)-FAIR. (_)-POOR... PROGRUSIS
(_)-GOOD. (_)-FAIR. (_)-POOR... HENABILITATION
POTENTIAL   (S-CPLEV)

(✓)-YES   (_)-NO........ RESIDENT IS AWARE OF
DIAGNOSIS, IF NO REASON:_____
(S-CPAWARE)

PRESCRIBER SIGNATURE _____   DATE _____
REVIEWED BY XXXXXXX   DATE 6/25/XX   NOTED BY _____   DATE _____

TOTAL RX: 0	TOTAL ROUTINES: 0	TOTAL PRN: 0
	TOTAL RTN TRMT: 0	TOTAL PRN TRMT: 0

*
*

REVIEW OF ENTIRE DRUG REGIMEN AND COMPREHENSIVE
RESIDENT CARE PLAN IS COMPLETED.
ANY IRREGULARITIES ARE DOCUMENTED IN THE
PHARMACIST'S MONTHLY REPORTS.
X
PHARMACY   DATE

☐ NO IRREGULARITIES NOTED
☐ INSIGNIFICANT IRREGULARITIES NOTED
☐ SIGNIFICANT IRREGULARITIES NOTED

☐ SEND * MEDS ONLY   ☐ SEND NO MEDS   ☐ SEND ALL MEDS

FIN PLAN-   SEX- M   DOB-
  NH RES#-   RES CODE- 96027

PRN, ORDERS

FIGURE 1-2.

© Apothesoft, LLC.

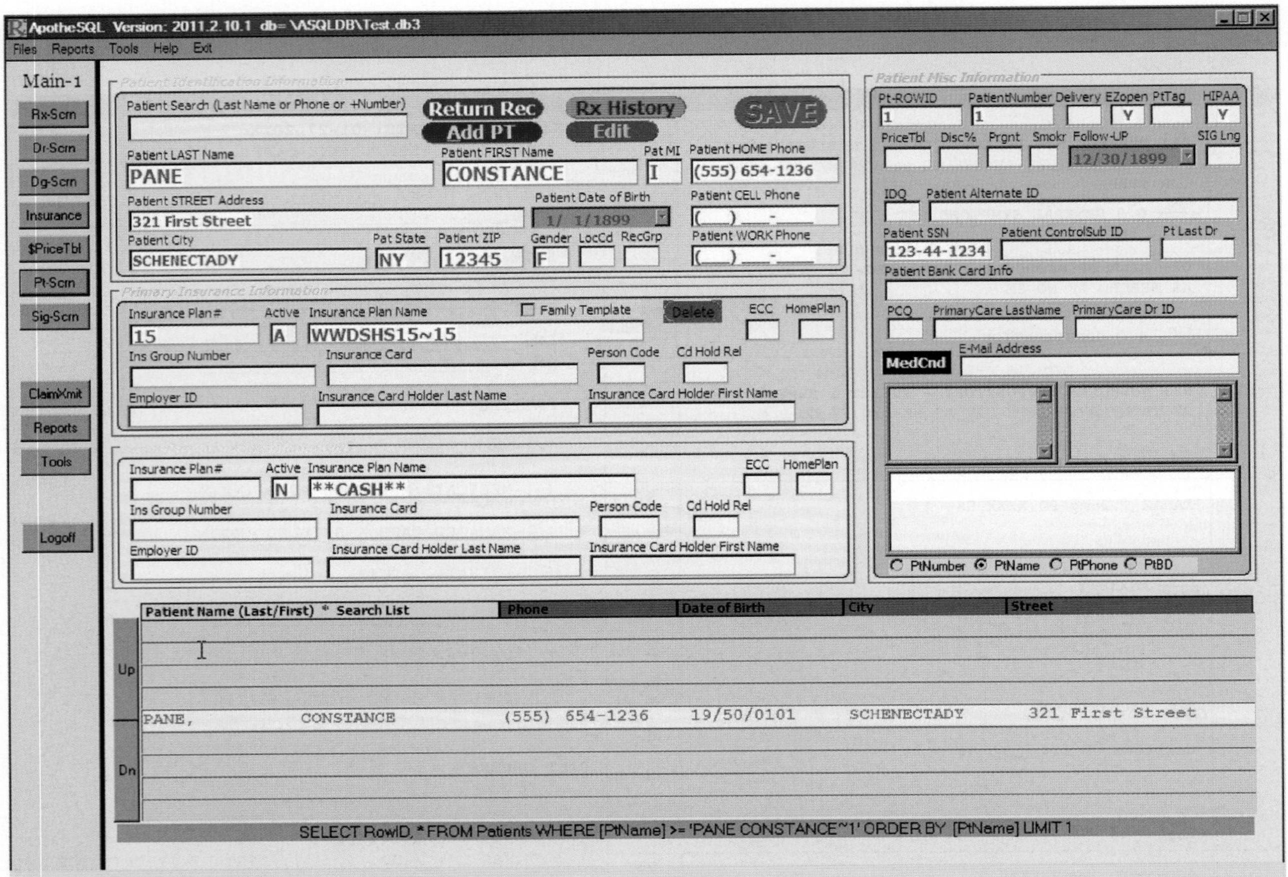

FIGURE 1-3.

© Apothesoft, LLC.

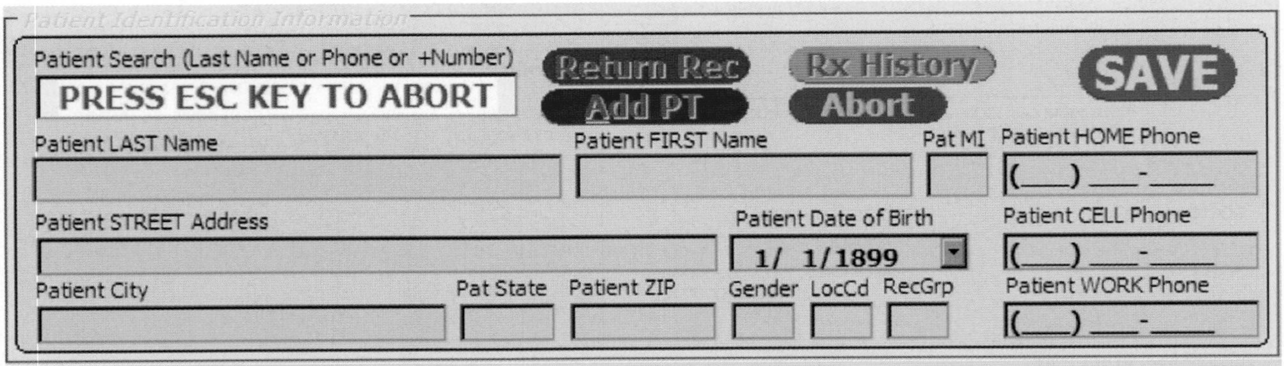

FIGURE 1-4.

© Apothesoft, LLC.

Adding a New Patient

To begin adding a new patient, click the button **Add PT** in the **Patient Identification Information** box. A new blank screen will appear. Enter the information in each blank space in the **Patient Identification Information** box (Figure 1-4). Advance from box to box using the ENTER or TAB key.

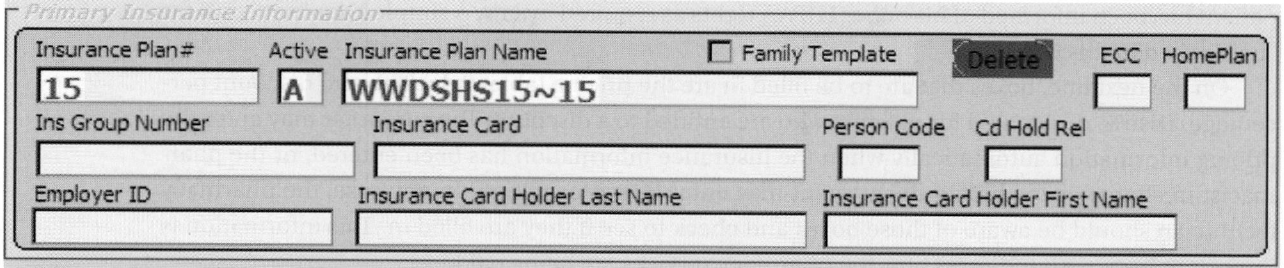

Primary Insurance Information

Insurance Plan#	Active	Insurance Plan Name	☐ Family Template	Delete	ECC	HomePlan

15 | A | WWDSHS15~15

Ins Group Number | Insurance Card | Person Code | Cd Hold Rel

Employer ID | Insurance Card Holder Last Name | Insurance Card Holder First Name

© Apothesoft, LLC.

FIGURE 1-5.

Secondary Insurance Information

Insurance Plan#	Active	Insurance Plan Name	ECC	HomePlan

0

Ins Group Number | Insurance Card | Person Code | Cd Hold Rel

Employer ID | Insurance Card Holder Last Name | Insurance Card Holder First Name

© Apothesoft, LLC.

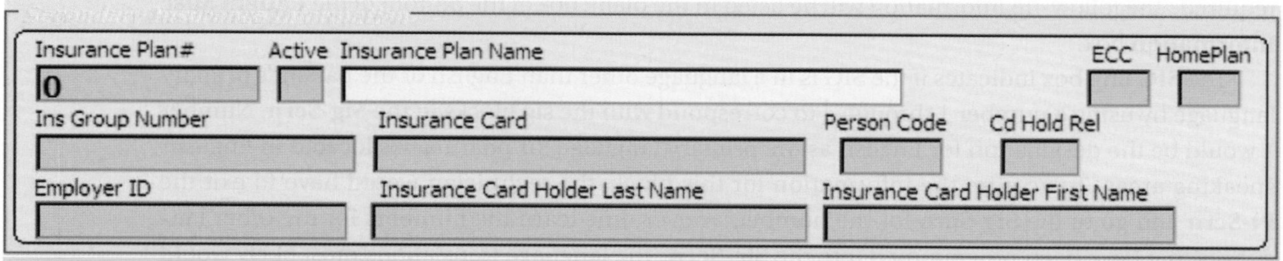

FIGURE 1-6.

After all the fields have been completed in the **Patient Identification Information** box, advance the cursor to **Primary Insurance Information** (Figure 1-5). Continue to hit **ENTER** or **TAB** until you have progressed through the **Primary Insurance Information** box. Entering patient insurance information will be discussed in detail in Chapter 4: Entering Insurance Claim Information.

After progressing all the way through the **Primary Insurance Information** box, the cursor will drop down to the **Secondary Insurance Information** box (Figure 1-6). Continue to **ENTER** or **TAB** through this box. After progressing through this box, the cursor will go to the **Patient Misc Information** box to the **Delivery** box (Figure 1-7).

The **Patient Misc Information** box captures additional information such as "gets prescriptions delivered or gets easy open vials." This information is entered in the box by a simple **Y** for "yes" or **N** for "no". The pharmacist assigns a two-letter designator, for a Skilled Nursing Facility or an assisted living facility, in the **PtTag** box. This box is used to pull all patients within a facility and print Medication Administration Reports (MARs) or simply print plain-paper reports for a hard-copy review of the patient's medications, allergies, medical conditions, and so forth. The next box, **HIPAA** (Healthcare Information Portability and Accountability Act), will show if the

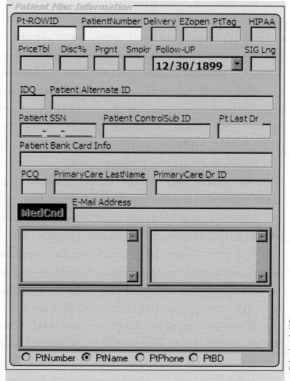

FIGURE 1-7.

patient has been informed of his or her HIPAA rights as required by law. A simple **Y** for "yes" or **N** for "no" is used in this box.

On the next line, boxes that are to be filled in are the pricing table, **PriceTbl**, and discount percentage, **Disc%**, designated for patients who are entitled to a discount. The computer may enter the pricing information automatically when the insurance information has been entered, or the pharmacist in charge or the billing department may enter this information. In any case, the pharmacy technician should be aware of those boxes and check to see if they are filled in. This information is important because it indicates how the pharmacy services are being paid.

In addition, some boxes are included to indicate whether the patient is pregnant (**Prgnt**) or is a smoker (**Smkr**); these are filled in with **Y** for "yes" and **N** for "no". The **Follow-UP** box indicates a date that will be referenced when pulling a report for patients for whom some type of follow-up is required. The follow-up information will be listed in the blank box at the bottom of the **Patient Misc Information** box.

The **SIG Lng** box indicates if the SIG is in a language other than English or the patient's primary language by using a number 1 through 4 to correspond with the sig blocks in the **Sig-Scrn**. Number 1 would be the designation for English as the primary language for pharmacies located in English-speaking areas. To acquire the information for this block, the technician would have to exit the **Pt-Scrn** and go to the **Sig-Scrn** for the number, or over time learn the numbers for the other languages that have been programmed into the **Sig-Scrn**. The language translations most likely would represent the prevalent languages in the immediate area surrounding the pharmacy.

Other boxes that have to be filled in are the identification qualifier (**IDQ**) for the patient and **Patient Alternate ID**. These fields are used for processing insurance and will be discussed in Chapter 4: Entering Insurance Claim Information.

The **Patient Misc Information** box gives the patient's Social Security number (**Patient SSN**), which is necessary for processing insurance claims. If this number is not entered correctly, the insurance claim may be rejected. Some states require information in the **Patient ControlSub ID** and **Pt Last Dr** boxes to track controlled substance use and thereby curtail abuse of prescription medications. The **Patient Bank Card Info** is used to allow for automatic billing of the patient's credit card.

Additional information boxes provide information such as the primary care qualifier (**PCQ**), primary care physician's last name, (**PrimaryCare LastName**), and the ID number (**PrimaryCare Dr ID**). These fields are all required for processing insurance claims, and the primary care physician's **E-Mail Address** for direct contact with the physician.

The **Pt-ROWID** and **PatientNumber**, at the top of the box, are generated by the software system after the patient information has been entered and saved. This information represents the position of the patient in the **Patient Name Search List**.

After all of the fields are complete, click on the **SAVE** button. A reminder box will pop up asking for you to OK the record to be saved (Figure 1-8).

Now that the record is saved, another reminder box will pop up to tell you that you must enter the patient's medical conditions and allergies (Figure 1-9).

After you click OK, the **Select Allergy & Medical Condition Codes for this Patient** screen will pop up for the appropriate information to be entered (Figure 1-10).

At the bottom of the block are two small boxes. The top box is checked and is labeled **Allergy Codes**. While this box is checked, you will be looking for the allergy codes by entering each of the patient's allergies in the box to the left of the **Find** button.

In the **Find** box, type in a search value for the patient's allergy. The search value may consist of a few letters or an ICD-9 code. The more complete the search value, the better and more defined the result will be. For example, if you type "ASA", the abbreviation for aspirin, into the search value box

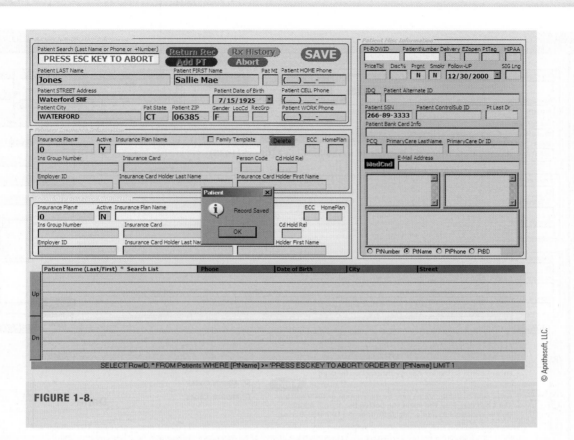

FIGURE 1-8.

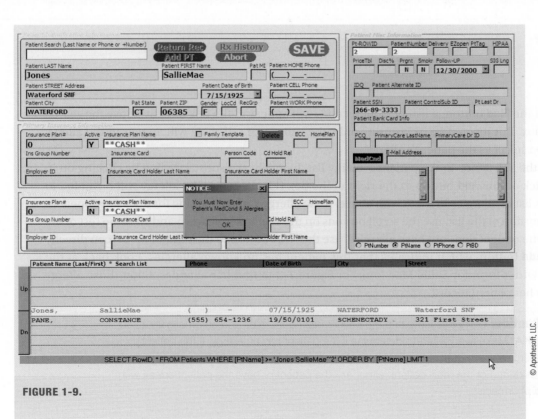

FIGURE 1-9.

© Apothesoft, LLC.

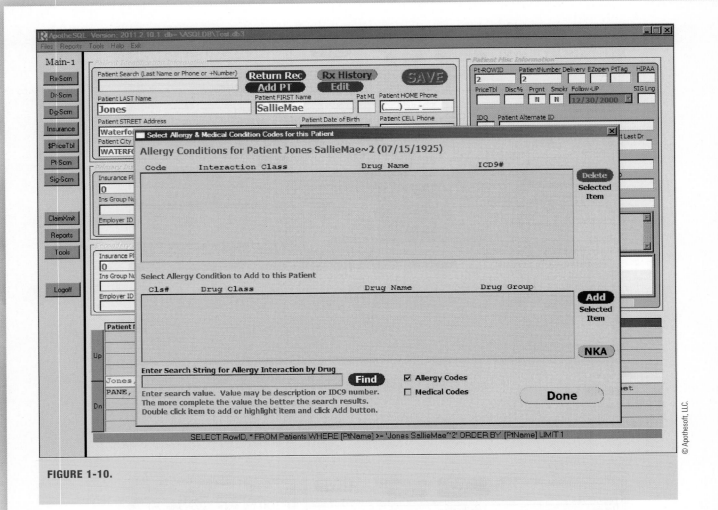

© Apothesoft, LLC.

FIGURE 1-10.

and click on the **Find** button, a listing of all A codes will appear in the box directly above the search value **Find** box. But if you type in "aspirin" only, the substance salicylate will appear in the allergy wcode box to select as the patient's allergy.

   To add the substance to the patient's allergy list, highlight the substance line by clicking on it, and then click on the **Add** button to the right of the box (Figure 1-11). The allergy will be added to the patient's list of allergies in the screen above. If the allergy you are looking for does not appear in the visible portion of the list, use the scroll buttons on the side to scroll down and view the rest of the list. Also, if the patient does not have allergies, use the **NKA** button to the right of the screen directly under the **Add** button, which indicates that this patient has no known allergies. Look back at the Physician's Order form for Sallie Mae Jones in Figure 1-2 to find her allergies. Enter those allergy notations in her patient record.

> **Caution:** Do not assume that the patient has no allergies and automatically select **NKA**. Make every effort to determine if the patient has an allergy. If the patient's allergies are in question, speak to the nurse at the facility where the patient is a resident. For the retail patient, either ask the patient or have the patient speak with a pharmacist.

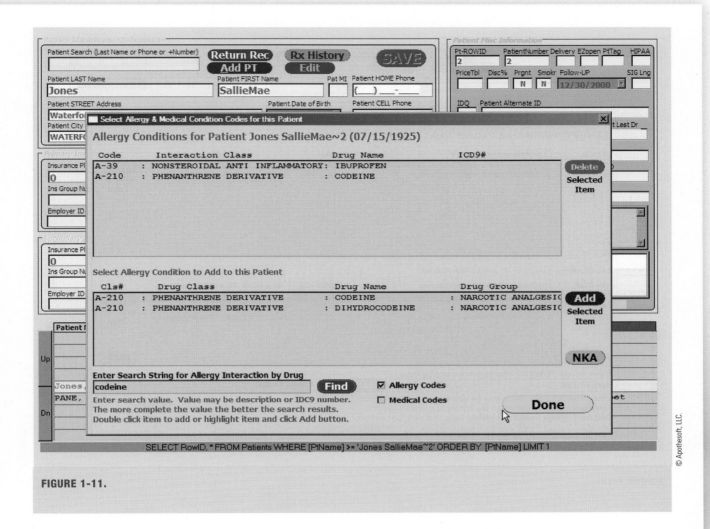

FIGURE 1-11.

Pharmacy technicians must understand the importance of entering allergy information correctly. When this is done, progress to entering the patient's medical conditions.

Check the box for **Medical Codes**, and in the **Find** box, type in a search value or ICD-9 code (Figure 1-12). Again, highlight the medical condition and click on the **Add** button. The condition will appear, along with the allergies in the list above. Enter the medical conditions for Sallie Mae Jones.

If an incorrect allergy or medical condition is entered, they are easily removed by highlighting the item to be removed and clicking on the **Delete** button.

Once you have entered in all of the patient's allergies and medical conditions, click on the **Done** button to return to the **Pt-Scrn**.

If the patient allergies or medical conditions are not found in the code lists, you can enter the information in the blank box at the bottom of the **Patient Misc Information** box.

Note: The allergy codes have an **A** as a prefix, and the medical codes have an **M** as a prefix.

Note: Before going to the next patient, take a few seconds to look over the information. If you see an error, correct it now by clicking on the **EDIT** button, making your correction, and clicking on the **SAVE** button again.

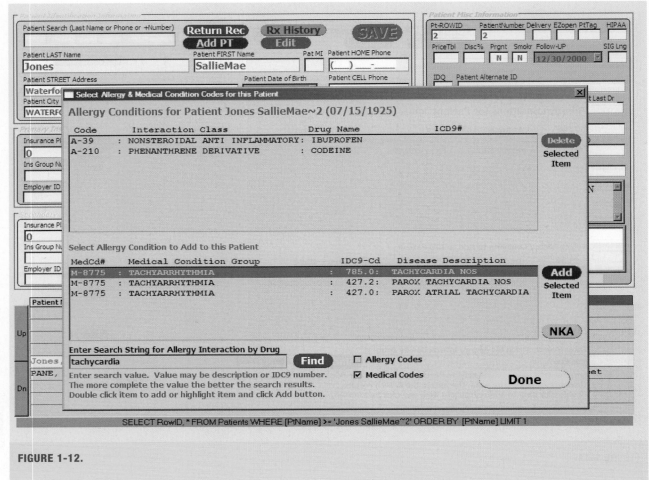

FIGURE 1-12.

Editing an Existing Patient

From time to time, changes will have to be made to the patient information. There are many reasons for editing a patient record. The first reason is correcting any mistakes made on initial input. The rest of the reasons will vary. The patient may have moved, changed telephone numbers, or changed physicians.

To make changes to a patient record, you must first find the correct patient. Once you have found the patient in **Pt-Scrn** by typing in the patient's last name in the **Patient Search** box. You will see the **Patient Name Search List** move to the patients with that last name. Select the right patient by using the up and down arrows or the mouse wheel. Check the screen to ensure you have the right patient. Check all of the information, address, Social Security number, physician, etc. Once you have determined that this is the correct patient, click on the **Edit** button and move to the correct box to make changes, corrections, or additions. When you are finished with editing the patient record, double-check your work and click on the **SAVE** button.

Note: Pharmacy technicians have to be both accurate and fast at entering all patient information into the computer. The pharmacist and the overall pharmacy operation depend upon that initial information entered into the pharmacy's computer system. As you complete the following exercises, try to increase your speed on each one, and check your accuracy as you increase your speed.

EXERCISE I

Create new patient profiles with the information provided below.

1. Patient: Mary Sue Wescott
    DOB: 4/19/1952
    Address: 1252 Summer Lane, Altamont, TN 37301
    Phone: 423-555-0100
    Cell: 423-555-0120
    SSN: 266-55-8888
    Doctor: William Jones, M.D.
    Allergies: Iodine
    Medical Condition: Depression

2. Patient: Robert S. Johnson
    DOB: 1/29/1938
    Address: 4568 Tumble Road, Cleveland, TN 37320
    Phone: 423-555-0124
    Cell: 423-555-0156
    SSN: 271-48-2020
    Doctor: Scott Smith, M.D.
    Allergies: NKA
    Medical Condition: None Listed

3. Patient: William Cakesmith
    DOB: 2/14/1950
    Address: 6723 West Liberty Street, Apison, TN 37302
    Phone: 423-555-0125
    Cell: 423-555-0157
    SSN: 201-22-8989
    Doctor: David Long, M.D.
    Allergies: Sulfa
    Medical Condition: Hypertension

4. Patient: Tommy Craig Holmes
    DOB: 7/19/1999
    Address: Waterford SNF, 2323 Lake Drive, Waterford, TN 37324
    Room: 23P
    Phone: 423-555-0197
    Cell:
    SSN: 212-28-3232
    Doctor: James Campbell, M.D.
    Allergies: NKA
    Medical Condition: Brain Damage

5. Patient: Judy Kay Wilson
   DOB: 8/30/1945
   Address: 9874 Horse Lane, Cleveland, TN 37312
   Phone: 423-555-0127
   Cell:
   SSN: 256-42-8989
   Doctor: William Jones, M.D.
   Allergies: Penicillin
   Medical Condition: Diabetes
6. Patient: Charles T. Cameron
   DOB: 7/18/1947
   Address: 895 Chamber Way, Apison, TN 37302
   Phone: 423-555-0126
   Cell: 423-555-0158
   SSN: 256-48-2412
   Doctor: Roger Lowell, M.D.
   Allergies: NKA
   Medical Condition: Hyperlipidemia

 Note: In the **Patient Misc Information** box, enter only the physician's last name in the **PrimaryCare LastName** box. You will build the physician's information in the **Dr-Scrn.**

EXERCISE II

Familiarity with the allergies list helps you enter the patient information and also helps you understand how the allergies are listed. Select a patient and click on the **Edit** button. In the **Patient Misc Information** box, click on the **MedCnd** button. The **Allergy Code & Medical Condition** box will pop up. Be sure that the **Allergy Codes** box is checked, and then enter the following allergies in the Search box and list the drug class for the allergy.

1. Cefoxitin
2. Valproic Acid
3. Amoxicillin
4. Phenytoin
5. Neomycin
6. Glyburide
7. Ciprofloxicin
8. Green Tea
9. Ranitidine
10. Naproxin

 Note: Type the name of the medication. When the drug appears, observe the listings under the headings Drug Class, Drug Name, and Drug Group. In observing the listings, you will become more familiar with the medications.

After you have entered the names of the above allergies, discuss the importance of listing the patient's allergies. If the allergies are not listed on the patient admission sheet or the prescription, how would you go about obtaining the patient's allergy information? If an allergy does not appear in the list, where would you list the allergy?

EXERCISE III

Becoming familiar with the medical conditions list allows you to enter the patient information more easily and also helps you understand how the medical conditions are listed and the many variations of a medical condition. These are listed because many medical conditions are associated with other medical complications. These associated conditions are significant to the prescriber and the pharmacist to ensure proper treatment and therapy. Insurance companies also require them for payment of a claim.

Select a patient, and click on the **Edit** button. In the **Patient Misc Information** box, click on the **MedCnd** button. The **Allergy Code & Medical Condition** box will pop up. Making sure that the **Medical Codes** box is checked, enter the following medical conditions in the **Find** box. To find the medical condition, scroll through the list for each medical condition to see the entire list, and select the one that is not associated with other medical conditions.

1. Hypothyroidism
2. Congestive Heart Failure (CHF)
3. Diabetes Mellitus Type II (DM)
4. Gout
5. Hypertension (HTN)
6. Mania (Bipolar)
7. Migraine
8. Porphyria
9. Chronic Obstructive Pulmonary Disease (COPD)
10. Asthma

 Note: When the abbreviation does not appear in the disease description, you must spell out the medical condition.

After you have entered the above medical conditions, discuss the importance of listing the patient's medical conditions. If the medical conditions are not listed on the patient admission sheet or on the prescription, how would you go about obtaining the patient's medical condition?

CRITICAL THINKING

1. What is the reason for entering as much patient information as possible?
2. Why is it necessary to know if the patient smokes?
3. Why should you know if the patient is pregnant?
4. What is the significance of entering the insurance information?
5. If the patient is in a nursing home, why should you make sure that the correct nursing home is entered in the **PtTag** box?
6. As a pharmacy technician, what is the significance of your role in ensuring that patient information is entered correctly in the computer?
7. Why should as many as possible of the patient's medical conditions be entered in the computer system?
8. Why should all of the patient's allergies be entered in the computer system?
9. Why is the patient's correct date of birth important?
10. Why should the middle initial of the patient be included?

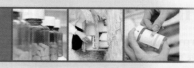

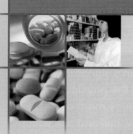

CHAPTER 2

Entering the Physician's Information

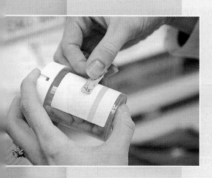

LEARNING OBJECTIVES

1. Describe the procedure for entering the physician information into the computer system.

2. Explain where additional physician information may be obtained.

3. Discuss the required physician information.

4. Point out the various types of physician license numbers that may be required for a physician to bill the patient insurance providers.

5. Explain how to edit the physician's information in the computer system.

This chapter explains how to enter a new physician into the pharmacy computer system as well as how to edit the physician information after it has been entered. The chapter also explains where additional physician information may be obtained if it is not available from the patient, prescription, or physician's order form. In addition, state licenses and Medicare and Medicaid licenses as discussed, and what the physician must do to obtain one of these licenses and who issues the licenses. The chapter concludes with a discussion of the **National Provider Identifier** number and the agency that issues the number to the physician.

As with the patient's information, discussed in Chapter 1, the physician's information must be accurate and complete. If it is not, problems will arise with insurance audits and billing for physicians and patients alike. As a pharmacy technician, your responsibilities include double-checking the information you enter in the computer system. If you receive information that you suspect or know is incorrect, you must check with the pharmacist. In no case should you change it yourself.

PHYSICIAN IDENTIFICATION INFORMATION

After entering the patient's information into the computer, pharmacy technicians must check to see if the patient's physician appears in the system. Look at the main screen. Navigate to the **Main-1** bar on the left side of the screen and click on **Dr-Scrn**. The **Doctor Identification Information** box will appear (Figure 2-1).

As you did with the patient, check to see if the physician is already entered in the system by typing in the physician's last name in the **Doctor Search** box. As a test, search for Scott Smith, M.D.—the doctor from the Skilled Nursing Facility on the Physician's Order form in Chapter 1 (Figure 1–1). You also could search for the physician

> **Note:** Sometimes a physician's signature is difficult to read, especially if the physician is working hastily in an emergency room or a clinic. In cases of uncertainty, call and ask which physician the patient saw, or ask the patient.

either by using the up and down arrows beside the names in the physician's **Search List** or typing the physician's telephone number in the **Doctor Search** box.

Once you have determined the physician's name, check the physician's telephone number and address. Sometimes you will run across more than one physician with the same last name or physicians working in several different locations.

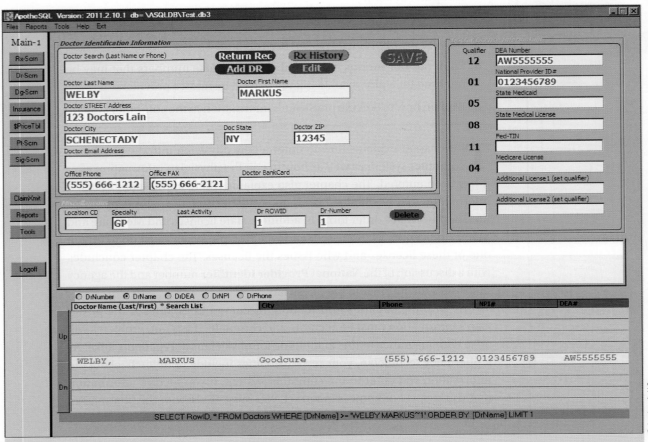

FIGURE 2-1.

© Apothesoft, LLC.

Entering a New Physician

If the physician is not in the system, click the button in the top center of the **Doctor Identification Information** box labeled **Add DR**. As a pharmacy technician, your responsibility is to ensure that the physician information is entered correctly in the system.

After clicking the **Add DR** button, a new blank screen will appear (Figure 2-2).

Enter the information requested in each blank box. Advance by using the `ENTER` key or the `TAB` key to move the cursor to the next empty box. After entering the **Doctor STREET Address**, `TAB` the cursor to the **Doctor ZIP** box, enter the zip code, and the computer will automatically fill in the **Doctor City** and **Doc State**. If the information inserted by the computer system is not correct, move back to the **Doctor City** box and enter the correct information.

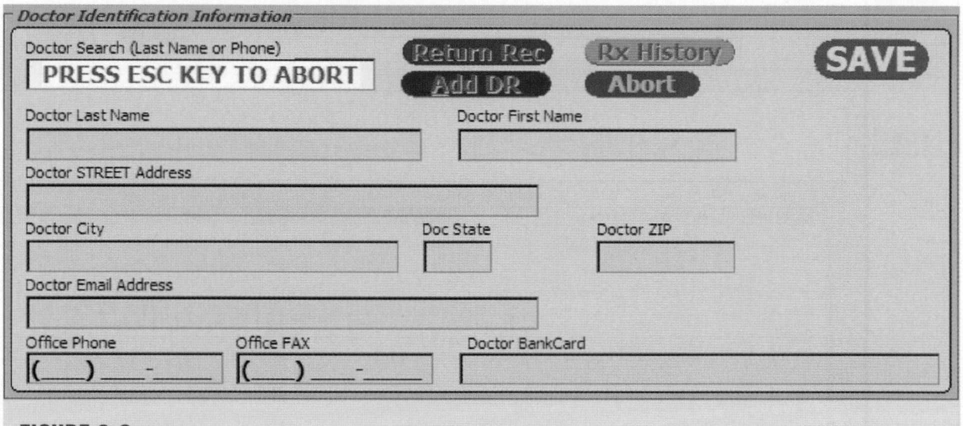

Note: Always double-check the spelling of both the first and last names of the physician. If information is missing as you proceed, contact the physician's office directly. Also check your state Department of Health professional licenses profiles on the Internet by typing in the Search box your state abbreviation and "DOH". At the Department of Health website, look for professional licenses profiles for the state.

FIGURE 2-2.

After all required information has been entered from **Doctor Last Name** to **Doctor BankCard**, pause and quickly look over the information before proceeding to the next block to ensure that the information is correct (Figure 2-3). *Entering accurate data in a timely manner is essential.*

Now enter the following information for Dr. Scott Smith:

```
Cardiologist
6456 Wayford Drive, Suite 101
Waterford, TN 37320
Phone: 423-555-0149
Fax: 423-555-0186
Email: heart2heart@smith.com
DEA#: 194590231
Medicaid #: 7578943
Medicare #: B41287
```

Note: The **BankCard** information is not required unless the physician wants to have an account with the pharmacy. This may not be included in other computer systems.

`TAB` or `ENTER` to the **Miscellaneous** block and enter in the information required in these fields if required by your pharmacy (Figure 2-4). The first box is the location code (**Location CD**). If your pharmacy operating system is managed by a corporate IT department, the computer may fill in this information automatically. If it is not managed in this way, the pharmacy might subscribe to a service that furnishes provider information to the pharmacy and updates the information for the pharmacy on a regular basis. An example of such a provider is HCIdea, a product of the National Council for Prescription Drug Programs (NCPDP), the website for which is *www.ncpdp.org*

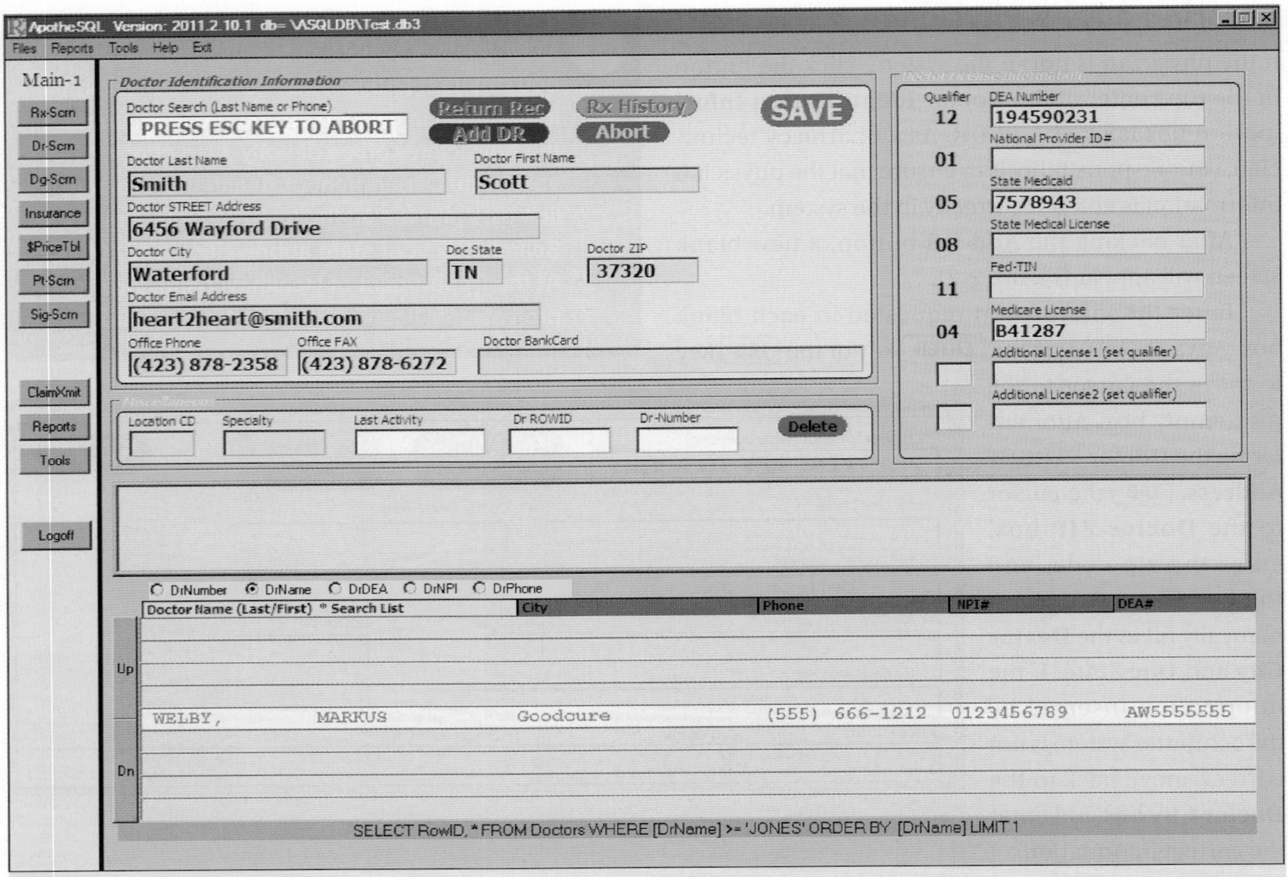

FIGURE 2-3.

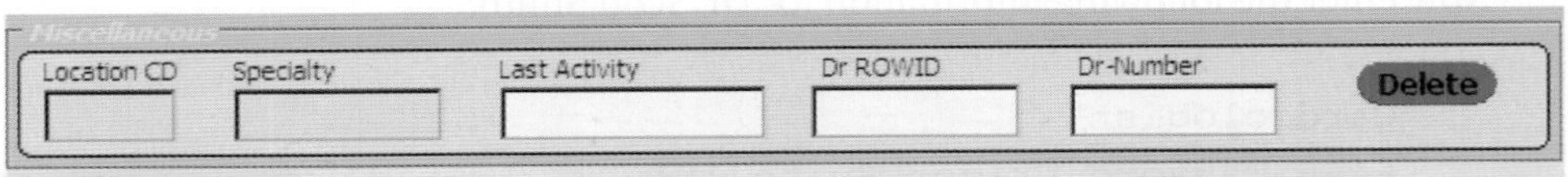

Next, ENTER or TAB over to the **Specialty** box, which indicates the physician's practice specialty or the type of provider, For example, 'PA' refers to Physician Assistant. The

FIGURE 2-4.

computer operating system may provide this information automatically. If it is not provided by an information service, it may be found in the heading of the prescription, or the yellow pages, or from the state Department of Health (DOH). The state DOH provides information on all licensed professionals who are working within the state.

The remaining boxes in the **Miscellaneous** box contain information related to the date of the provider's **Last Activity** with the pharmacy, which is generated by the computer and the location, **Dr ROWID** and **Dr-Number**, of the provider in the **Search List**.

> **Note:** NPPES, the National Plan and Provider Enumeration System, was developed by the Center for Medicare and Medicaid Services (CMS) for administration simplification provisions of the Health Insurance Portability and Accountability Act of 1996 (HIPAA), which mandates the adoption of a unique identifier for health care providers. You can search for provider information on the NPPES website *https://nppes.cms.hhs.gov*

© Apothesoft, LLC.

The **Doctor License Information** box starts with the **Qualifier 12** (Figure 2-5). Qualifier 12 is a prescriber ID qualifier that corresponds to the prescriber's **DEA number**.

The qualifier numbers are two-digit codes that designate required information in a short-form code. These qualifiers are used when processing insurance claims. The computer system will retrieve the information from this **Doctor License Information** box when the qualifier number is entered in the appropriate box in the insurance processing screens.

For each of the qualifiers in the **Doctor License Information** box, you will enter a number that has been issued to that provider through a national or state organization or government agency. The **Qualifier 01** is the **National Provider ID #** (NPI), a unique 10-digit identification number issued to health care providers in the United States by the Centers for Medicare and Medicaid Services (CMS). The **National Provider ID #** (NPI) must be used in connection with the electronic transactions identified in HIPAA. The **NPI** is used by health care providers on prescriptions (the NPI, however, will not replace requirements for the Drug Enforcement Administration number or State license number).

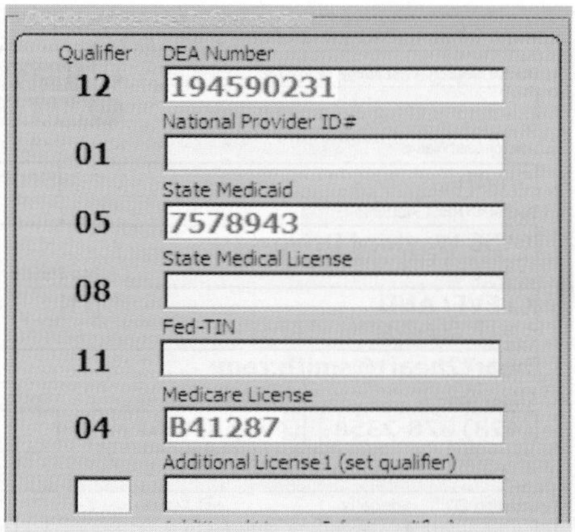

The **Qualifier 05** is the **State Medicaid** provider number issued to the states through the Centers for Medicare and Medicaid Services' Department of Health and Human Services to the State Health and Human Service agencies. The Medicaid provider numbers are issued to physicians or other providers who apply to their state issuing agency. If physicians do not accept Medicaid, they would not have a Medicaid number.

The **Qualifier 08** is the **State Medical License** number issued to the provider by the State Medical Board after completion of state licensing requirements. The **Qualifier 11** is the **Fed-TIN** (Federal Tax Identification Number), the tax identification number issued by the Internal Revenue Service to the provider. Finally, the **Qualifier 04** is the **Medicare License** number issued by the Centers for Medicare and Medicaid Services (CMS). To receive the number, the provider first must apply for a **National Provider Identifier** (NPI) and then, after receiving an NPI number, complete an application for the **Medicare License** from CMS.

Qualifier DEA Number
12 194590231
National Provider ID #
01
State Medicaid
05 7578943
State Medical License
08
Fed-TIN
11
Medicare License
04 B41287
Additional License 1 (set qualifier)

© Apothesoft, LLC.

FIGURE 2-5.

Note: Chapter 4 addresses the manual verification of DEA numbers.

Note: If the computer system does not provide this information automatically from an information provider, you can look up the NPI number at the NPI Lookup website, *www.npinumberlookup.org*

Note: If you have to add information about the provider, in free form, to the screen, you can click on the blank box in the center of the screen and add comments before saving the screen information.

Note: Be sure to check the changes for accuracy before saving the information.

Two blank qualifier boxes allow for any additional information that may be required by the pharmacy for which you are working for or the state in which your pharmacy is located.

Once the **Doctor License Information** box is complete, look over the information to verify that all of the information is correct, and then click on the **SAVE** button at the top of the screen. The physician's information now will appear in the doctor's directory and will appear in the **Search List** (Figure 2-6).

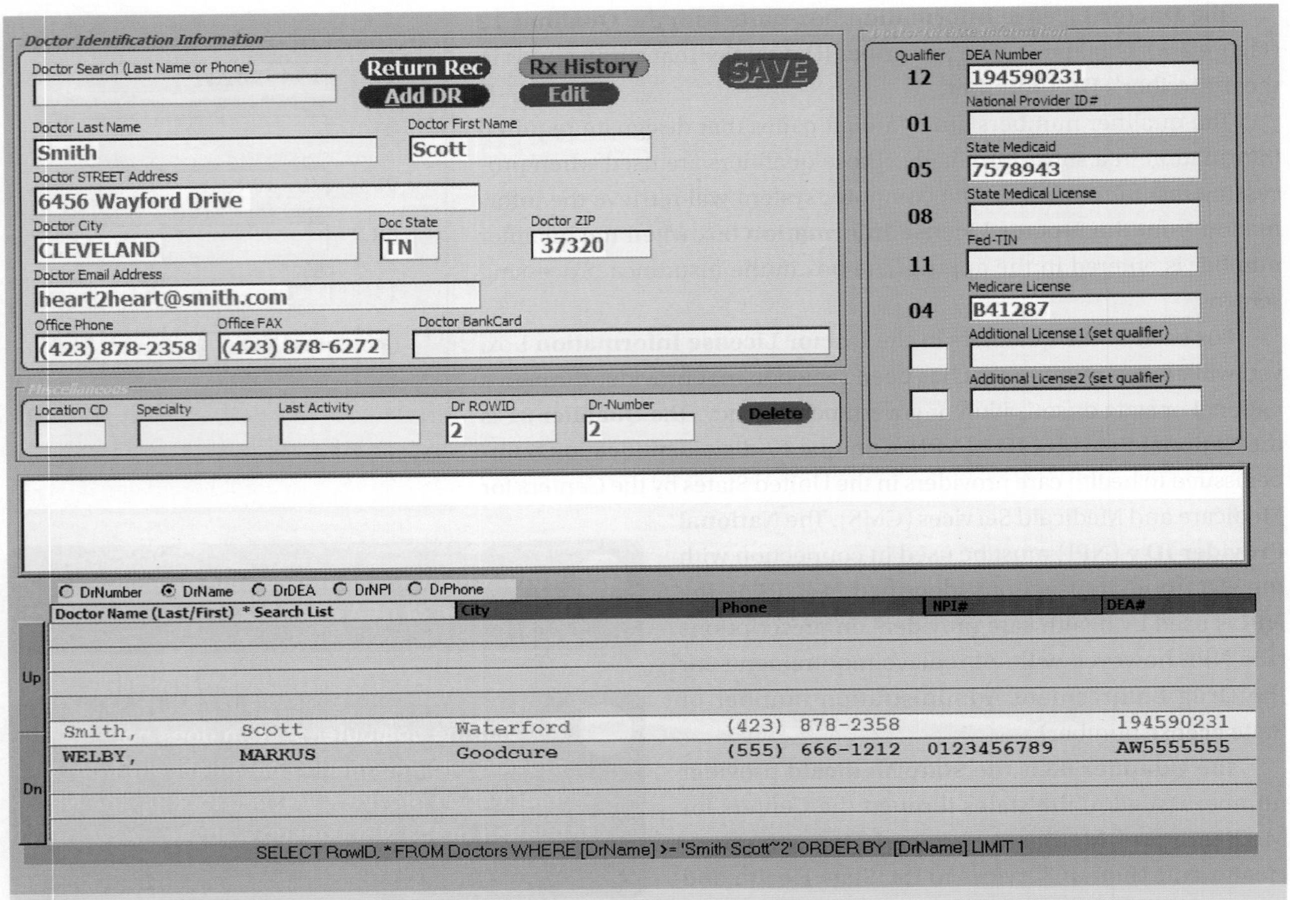

FIGURE 2-6.

Editing an Existing Physician

From time to time, changes will have to be made to the physician's information. Errors may have occurred on the initial input of this information, the physician may have moved his or her office, or the physician may have additional qualifiers to be added to the information.

Whatever the reason for making changes, simply click on the **Edit** button in the **Dr-Scrn** and make the changes, then click on the **SAVE** button.

EXERCISE I

Create new doctor profiles with the information provided below.

```
1. James Campbell, MD
   Pediatrician
   2345 Waycross Drive
   Collegedale, TN 37315
   Phone: 423-555-0141
   Fax: 423-555-0196
   Email: kidsplace@james.net
```

DEA #: AC2345676
NPI: 1930183128
Medicaid #: 5438965

2. William Jones, MD.
   Neurologist
   6456 Wayford Drive Suite 200
   Waterford, TN 37320
   Phone: 423-555-0153
   Fax: 423-555-0184
   Email: neurospecialities@turner.net
   DEA #: BJ1323561
   NPI: 1930393137
   Medicaid #: 5438687
   Medicare #: B60602

3. David Long, MD
   General Practitioner
   6456 Wayford Drive Suite 300
   Waterford, TN 37320
   Phone: 423-555-0142
   Fax: 423-555-0195
   Email: healthplace@long.net
   DEA #: BL1325489
   NPI: 1931395623
   Medicaid #: 5456894
   Medicare #: B60735

4. Roger Daniel Lowell, MD
   Gastroenterologist
   3510 Kimmons Street Suite B
   Calhoun, TN 37309
   Phone: 423-555-0152
   Fax: 423-555-0194
   Email: mattersofthegut@daniel.com
   DEA #: AL2486579
   NPI: 1930395489
   Medicaid #: 5465687
   Medicare #: B61856

5. Jane Smith, DO
   Internal Medicine Specialist
   6456 Wayford Drive Suite 100
   Waterford, TN 37320
   Phone: 423-555-0147
   Fax: 423-555-0185
   Email: wellnessclinic@smith.com
   DEA #: BS2568972
   NPI: 193653289
   Medicaid #: 5436598
   Medicare #: B61882

```
6. Thomas Frye, DO
   Cardiologist
   5561 Westfield Circle
   Calhoun, TN 37309
   Phone: 423-555-0148
   Fax: 423-555-0193
   Email: waterfordheart@thomas.net
   DEA #: AF1356498
   NPI: 1930564623
   Medicaid #: 5437799
   Medicare #: B60403
```

EXERCISE II

Select at least six physicians in your area and look up the information for each of them on the following websites. Print out the information on each physician.

1. Your state Department of Health (DOH)

2. *www.npinumberlookup.org*

3. *https://nppes.cms.hhs.gov*

EXERCISE III

Discuss the importance of knowing what type of provider is writing the prescription for the medication. What do you know about your state's laws covering various provider prescribing permissions?

CRITICAL THINKING

1. What is the importance of your entering as much information as possible about the physician ?

2. Why are notes entered into the Note section of the Miscellaneous block?

3. Why does the DEA number have to be entered correctly?

4. Why does the **National Provider Identifier** information have to be accurate?

5. On which occasions, if any, may a provider not be allowed to write for controlled substances?

6. What is the importance of your entering the correct provider information in the computer?

7. Why should you enter the provider's e-mail address, and what other information would be useful to enter in the Notes?

8. How would you handle a prescription, written or printed, on which multiple providers are printed at the top, you are unable to read the signature, and the provider's name is not checked, circled, or underlined?

9. What is the importance of an accurate state Medicaid provider number?

10. Why do think the middle initial of the provider might constitute essential information?

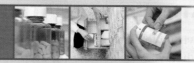

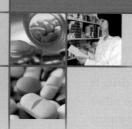

CHAPTER 3

Inputting Inventory

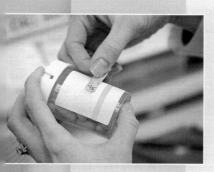

LEARNING OBJECTIVES

1. Emphasize the importance of checking the computer before entering a drug into the computer.

2. Define the purpose of the National Drug Code number.

3. Enumerate the components of the NDC number.

4. Explain the difference between the UPC number and the NDC number.

5. Discuss the importance of using a company such as Lexi-Comp.

6. Explain the meanings of AAC, AWP, and MAC.

An inventory consists of all the items maintained in the pharmacy that are needed for pharmacy operation. In addition to medications, the inventory includes medical supplies, dispensing supplies, and office supplies. Maintaining inventory is an essential, detail-oriented job within the pharmacy. It requires knowledge of *how* to enter the products into the computer and also *what* is needed. The responsible pharmacy purchaser also must be familiar with all of the sources of supplies and costs associated with those supplies. This chapter explains how to input medications into the pharmacy's computer.

Supplies and inventories of medication have to be kept up-to-date and monitored at all times. The inventory may be updated by a pharmacist or a pharmacy technician at the local level or by the IT department at the pharmacy's corporate headquarters. The pharmacy technician may be responsible for maintaining the pharmacy inventory and may be asked at some time to enter a new inventory item for a prescription to be filled or processed.

DRUG IDENTIFICATION INFORMATION

To begin to enter inventory, navigate to the drug screen (**Dg-Scrn**) button under the **Main-1** bar on the left side of the screen. When you click on the **Dg-Scrn** button, the drug screen will appear (Figure 3-1).

After accessing the **Dg-Scrn** and before entering a new drug or compound, scroll through the drug list to ensure that the drug is not in the system already. Using the up and down arrows on the left side of the list or using the mouse wheel, scroll through the drug list to determine if the drug is in the inventory in that specific strength, form, or size of container. This list also includes the other inventory supply items in the pharmacy, such as alcohol pads, syringes with needles, intravenous tubing, intravenous pumps, and adult diapers.

To check for the drug more rapidly than by scrolling, type the drug name, the first few letters of the drug or NDC (National Drug Code number) in the **Drug Search** box. After typing the name, you will see the first few letters of the drug or supply item, or NDC number, and the **Search List** will move to that item, highlighted in red.

Long-term care pharmacies and institutional pharmacies house more supply items than retail pharmacies do. The pharmacy technician is responsible for maintaining these medications on the shelves as well as the operational supplies and unique supplies needed by individual patients.

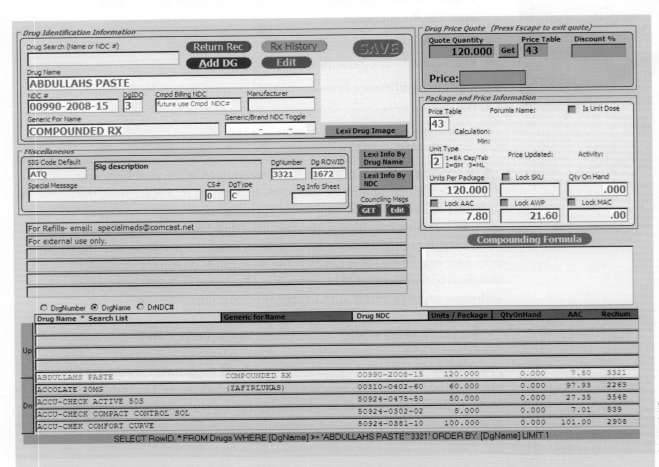

FIGURE 3-1.

© Apothesoft, LLC.

Once you have determined if you have or do not have the drug or supply item in the inventory, proceed with the appropriate action. If the drug is in the system already, you may have to add a different size, form, or strength. If you do not find the drug or supply item you are looking for, you will have to enter all of the required information for that drug or supply item.

ENTERING A NEW DRUG OR SUPPLY ITEM

Search for the drug **SANCUSO** to determine if this medication exists in the pharmacy inventory. As you enter **SAN** into the **Drug Search** box, the drug list will move to the drugs, starting with the letter "S." The **Search List** shows that **SANCUSO** has not been entered in the computer system inventory (Figure 3-2).

To begin entering a new drug or supply item into the computer system inventory, be sure that you have all the information about the drug or supply item. You will have to gather all the information requested in the **Drug Identification Information** box. Two particularly helpful pieces of information are the item and the supplier's invoice, which will give you most, if not all, of the information you need. Accessing this information will save you time, and entering a new drug will be much easier and error free.

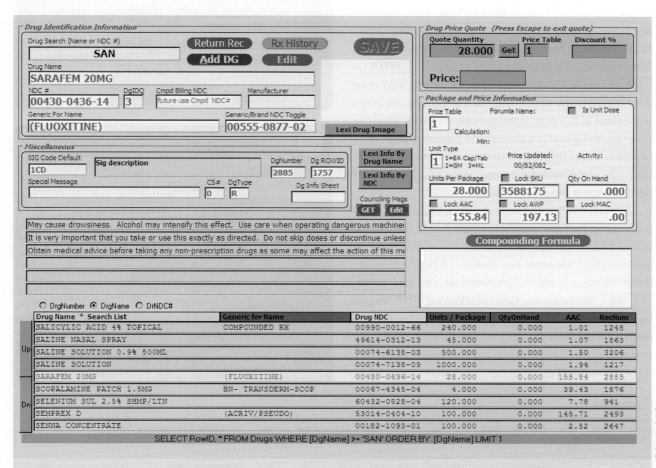

FIGURE 3-2.

© Apothesoft, LLC.

At the top of the **Drug Identification Information** box, close to the middle of the screen, you will find the **Add DG** button. After you click on it, the screen will clear all the information from the boxes in the screen in preparation for the new drug or supply item information. Type the name of the drug or supply item in the **Drug Name** box, and *double-check to make sure that it is spelled correctly*. Now `ENTER` or `TAB` to the **NDC #** box and enter the NDC number.

If you are entering a supply item, use the Universal Product Code (UPC) bar code on the product. The UPC code is different from the NDC number. It has 11 digits instead of 10 as the primary product identifier and a 12th digit, which serves as a "check digit" that tells the scanner that the number is correct or incorrect. The scanner performs a mathematical calculation to check against the 12th digit and verify the product.

After you have entered the NDC number or UPC code, hit `ENTER` or `TAB`. Notice that the cursor skipped over the **Cmpd Billing NDC** box. This box will be used later when entering a compound. At the **Manufacturer** box, enter the manufacturer's name. After entering the manufacturer's name hit `ENTER` or `TAB` to get to the **Generic For Name** box and enter the generic name of the drug. In most cases, the active ingredient in the drug is the generic name for the drug. Entering the generic name inside parentheses is good practice, as an indication that the first name appearing in the drug list is the brand name and the name in parentheses is the generic name.

When scrolling through the drug list, notice that if the generic name of a drug is listed first in the list, the brand name will appear without parentheses in the column titled **Generic For Name**. After you have entered the generic name, **Granisetron**, and hit `ENTER` or `TAB`, move to the **Generic/Brand NDC Toggle** box. This box will have the NDC number for the **Generic** or **Brand,** depending on which was listed in the first box of the **Drug Information Identification** box. If you have listed the generic name in the **Drug Name**

Note: The NDC (National Drug Code) number serves as a universal product identifier for human drugs. The Drug Listing Act of 1972 requires that all registered drug manufacturers provide the Food and Drug Administration (FDA) with a current list of their manufactured drugs, preparations, compounds, and processes they distribute for commercial purposes. Each NDC number is assigned a unique 10-digit, 3-segment number. The number identifies the labeler, product, and package size. The first segment identifies the manufacturing firm (including repackers or relabelers) or distributors of the drug. The second segment identifies the product's strength, dosage form, and formulation for the specific firm. The third segment identifies the package sizes and types. The NDC will be configured in a 4-4-2 or 5-3-2 or 5-4-1 number pattern. The NDC number is a 10-digit number, and an asterisk (*) will appear as a place holder in some numbers. Also, the HIPAA standard of an 11-digit NDC requires that many programs use a leading zero (0) instead of an asterisk in the package or product code. Table 3-1 shows examples of NDC configurations for a drug product.

Note: The UPCs are originated by the Uniform Code Council (UCC) company, which, for an annual fee, supplies the manufacturer with an identification number and guidelines explaining how to use it. The first six digits of the UPC code designate the manufacturer, the next five digits represent the product, and the last digit is the check number. The number 3 as the first digit designates that the product is a pharmaceutical (Figure 3-3). Shorter UPCs are known as zero-suppressed numbers. The zeros in the numbers have been suppressed, and only the manufacturer and product digits are shown along with the check number.

TABLE 3:1

Product Trade Name	NDC Code (5-4-2)	NDC Code (5-4-1/ 5-3-2)	NDC Code (541/532)	NDC Code (542)	Labeler Code	Product Code	Package Code	RX/OTC	Package Size	Package Type	Active Ingredients	Routes of Administration	Dosage Form	Strength	Unit Of Measure
ABILIFY TABLETS	15548 -*00713	15548 -00713	1554800713	15548000713	15548	*007	13	R	30	BOT	ARIPIPRAZOLE 5 MG	ORAL	TABLET	5	MG

Example of NDC number in different segments

© Cengage Learning 2012

box and its NDC number in the **NDC #** box, you will list the brand name in the **Generic For Brand** box and the brand's NDC number (Figure 3-4). Once the NDC number has been entered, hit ENTER or TAB and the cursor will move to the **Miscellaneous** box and the **SIG Code Default** box.

The **Miscellaneous** box contains the **SIG Code Default** box and the **Sig description** box, which will show the translation of the **SIG Code Default** after the information has been entered in **Sig-Scrn** (discussed later). Pharmacists at times ask pharmacy technicians to help enter the sig codes and the sig descriptions. If so, the code should be easy to remember or easy to look up, especially if it is a sig, which is specific for a given drug. As always, check with the pharmacist to be sure the information is correct.

The **SIG Code Default** is the short code that enables you to enter prescriptions faster. For example, the SIG code **1PD24H** is much faster and easier to type than **Use one patch daily for 24 hours before chemotherapy; remove 24 hours after**

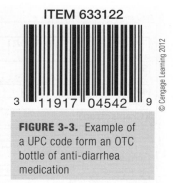

© Cengage Learning 2012

ITEM 633122

3 11917 04542 9

FIGURE 3-3. Example of a UPC code form an OTC bottle of anti-diarrhea medication

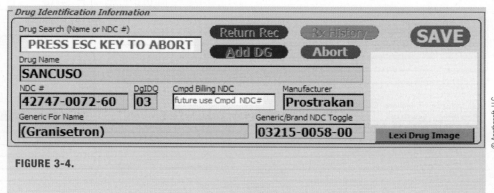

Drug Identification Information

Drug Search (Name or NDC #)
PRESS ESC KEY TO ABORT   Return Rec   Rx History   SAVE
                            Add DG   Abort

Drug Name
SANCUSO

NDC #   DgIDQ   Cmpd Billing NDC   Manufacturer
42747-0072-60   03   future use Cmpd NDC#   Prostrakan

Generic For Name   Generic/Brand NDC Toggle
(Granisetron)   03215-0058-00   Lexi Drug Image

© Apothesoft, LLC.

FIGURE 3-4.

chemotherapy. The expanded wording will appear on the printed label to be placed on the medication that is dispensed to the patient.

After entering the SIG Code default, hit ENTER or TAB, and the cursor will skip over the **DgNumber** and **DgROWID**, which shows the location of the drug in the **Search List**, and move to the **Special Message** box. In this case, the message **Apply to upper arm** is entered because this is the recommended site for placing the patch.

Hit ENTER or TAB and move to the next box, **CS#**, which stands for Controlled Substance schedule number. Because Sancuso is not a controlled substance, a "0" will be entered in the box. After entering "CS#", hit ENTER or TAB and move to the **DgType** box. This box designates if a drug is a regular legend drug requiring a prescription, which can be designated by an **R**, or a non-legend OTC, which does not require a prescription, designated by **O**. (Some pharmacies use other codes.)

Hit ENTER or TAB and move to the **Dg Info Sheet** box, which will indicate if this drug or item has a drug information sheet. *Always check the information for correctness and completeness before moving to the next box* (Figure 3-5).

To enter counseling messages, click on the **Edit** button under **Counciling Msgs**. A drop down box, **Select Drug Messages**, will appear with a list of messages that may be checked and selected to add to the counseling information for the drug (Figure 3-6). If you have to remove a message, right-click on the line to be deleted, and a delete box will pop up. Click **OK**. After entering the information in the **Miscellaneous** box, double-check to make sure that the information is correct before moving to the next section.

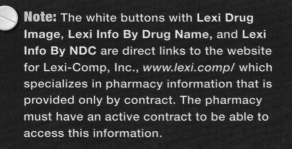

Note: The white buttons with **Lexi Drug Image, Lexi Info By Drug Name,** and **Lexi Info By NDC** are direct links to the website for Lexi-Comp, Inc., *www.lexi.comp/* which specializes in pharmacy information that is provided only by contract. The pharmacy must have an active contract to be able to access this information.

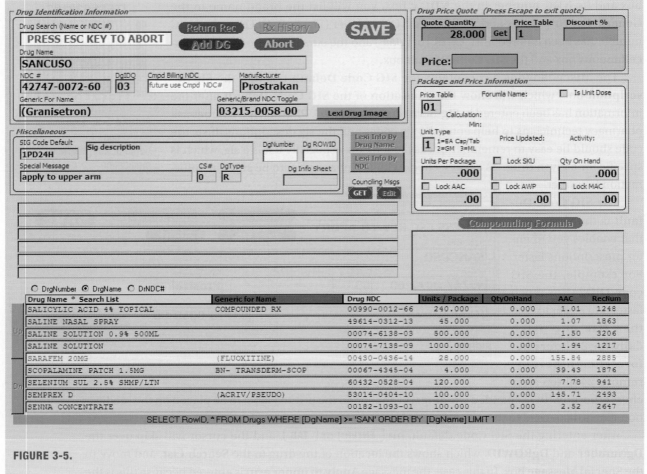

FIGURE 3-5.

ENTER or TAB over to the **Price Table** box inside the **Package and Price Information** box (Figure 3-7). This information must be completed before the drug can be saved so the information will appear in the computer system's **Search List**. The first box, **Price Table**, is extremely important. The price table number indicates which formula for pricing is being used from the **Price** Table, which may be accessed by selecting the **$PriceTbl** button on left side of screen under **Main-1**. In this case, we are using Price Table 2.

If the pharmacy technician is required to enter new drugs or supply items, certain guidelines must be followed concerning the pricing of each item that will go into the inventory. *The pricing, if not completed correctly, will affect the pharmacy revenue.*

After entering the price information, click on the **Unit Type** box and select how the drug will be dispensed. If the drug is in a capsule or tablet form, enter **1** for **EA** (each). This asks for dispensing the unit as one tablet or capsule. If the drug is measured in either **GM** (grams) or **ML** (milliliters) enter the corresponding number. Next enter the **Units Per Package**, which refers to the number of units in one package. For example, if you have entered 1 for EA and a package contains only one patch per box, you would enter 1.000; then ENTER or TAB over to **Qty On Hand**. Quantity on hand refers to the physical inventory in stock or on the shelf. If there are three boxes on the shelf, you would enter "3" for the quantity in the pharmacy.

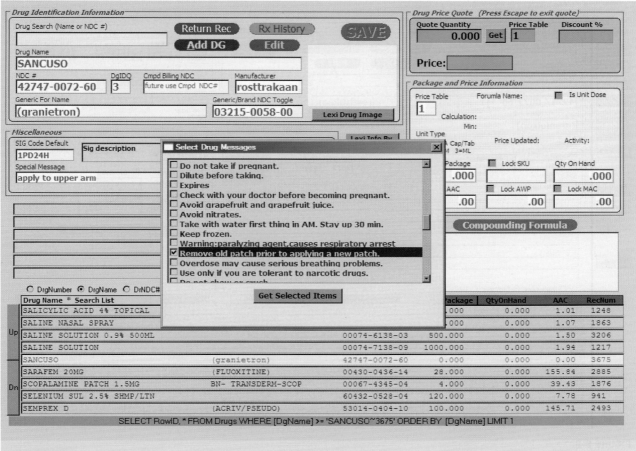

© Apothesoft, LLC.

FIGURE 3-6.

Next enter the acquisition cost for the package in the **AAC** box. The acquisition cost will appear on the order invoice or in the software provided by the wholesale distributor. This information is used to calculate the pricing for each unit that will be dispensed by the pharmacy.

The next box is for the **AWP** (Average Wholesale Price), the average price for which a wholesaler will sell drugs to pharmacies. If the AWP is used to calculate the drug price, the AWP cost usually is discounted by an allowed or negotiated percentage. The AWP most often is the cost used to calculate the allowable reimbursement for health insurance. The pricing is based on a formula consisting of the AWP minus a percentage plus a dispensing fee.

The next box is the **MAC** (Maximum Allowable Cost), which is used to set the upper-limit prices that a health plan will pay. Typically, when this price is entered, it is set by reimbursements

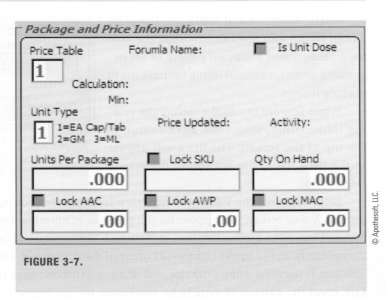

FIGURE 3-7.

© Apothesoft, LLC.

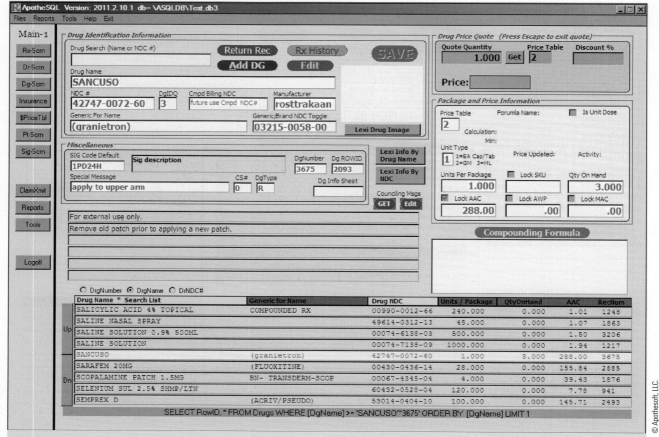

FIGURE 3-8.

allowed by Medicare and Medicaid. This price would be set and used to calculate the cost for a Medicare or Medicaid patient or for negotiated costs for certain items for patients in nursing homes.

When you are finished entering the pricing information, select the **SAVE** button at the top of the screen. The drug will appear in the drug list at the bottom of the screen (Figure 3-8).

FIGURE 3-9.

Directly below the **Package and Price Information** box appears a **Compounding Formula** button. A new screen will appear for the purpose of entering the ingredients needed to make a requested compound when this button is clicked. This screen will be discussed in Chapter 6: Inputting Compounds. In the upper righthand corner of the screen is the **Drug Price Quote** box (Figure 3-9). This box is used for estimating the cost of a prescription. After selecting the drug from the **Search List**, enter the amount of drug to be dispensed, the pricing table number, and any discount. When you click on the **Get** button, the computer will calculate the cost of the prescription. Most computer systems allow for estimating costs to quote to a patient or customer. This question is asked of pharmacy personnel frequently, and the patient or customer expects a quick and courteous answer.

EXERCISE I

You have received a shipment of drugs and removed the invoice from the tote. Now you have to enter the drugs into the pharmacy system. Before doing so, check the **DgScrn Search List**. Are these drugs in the computer already? If not, you will have to enter them. Check the drug labels against the invoice. If the labels match the invoice and the drugs are not in the computer, enter them.

DRUG WHOLESALER
INVOICE

BILL TO	Your Pharmacy 4568 Drug Court Suite B Birchwood, TN 37345	SHIP TO	Your Pharmacy 4568 Drug Court Suite B Birchwood, TN 37345	Invoice # 456888
				Invoice Date 10/25/20XX
				Customer ID 12369

DATE	YOUR ORDER #	OUR ORDER #	SALES REP.	F.O.B.	SHIP VIA	TERMS	TAX ID
10/25	897	2301	MW			Net 30	5668-896-89

QTY	NDC#	UNITS	DESCRIPTION	DISCOUNT %	TAXABLE	UNIT PRICE	TOTAL
3	0078-0458-05	100	Lopressor 50 mg	3		198.32	594.96
2	0008-1211-14	14	Prestiq 50 mg	5		145.35	290.70
4	0088-1102-47	100	Allegra 60 mg	3		215.50	862.00
1	0048-1020-05	1000	Synthroid 25 mcg	5		921.90	921.90
5	0071-0418-24	100	Nitrostat 0.4 mg	6		88.66	443.30
2	18393-272-62	500	Naprosyn 250 mg	3		90.00	180.00
4	0378-5012-01	100	Felodipine Extended Release 5 mg	8		131.70	526.80
3	0378-6400-01	100	Erythromycin 400 mg	10		135.52	406.56
6	0039-0067-50	500	Lasix 20 mg	10		47.40	284.40
3	0083-0052-30	100	Tergretol 100 mg	3		60.00	180.00

Subtotal	4690.62
Tax	
Shipping	
Miscellaneous	
BALANCE DUE	$4690.62

© Cengage Learning 2012

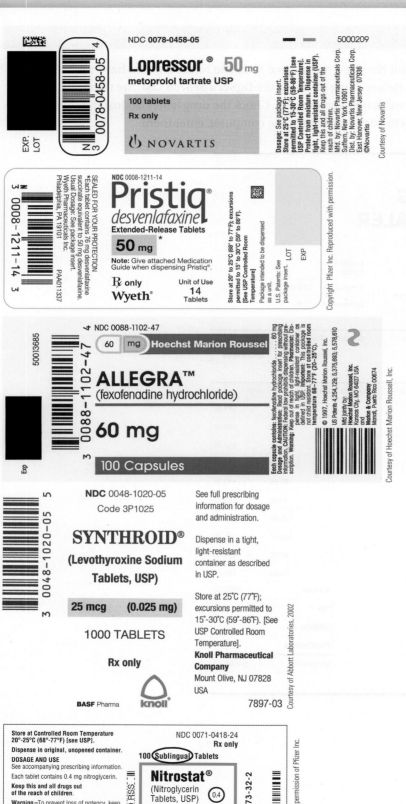

NDC 0078-0458-05

Lopressor ® 50 mg

metoprolol tartrate USP

100 tablets

Rx only

ᘉ **NOVARTIS**

5000209

Dosage: See package insert.
Store at 25°C (77°F); excursions
permitted to 15-30°C (59-86°F) [see
USP Controlled Room Temperature].
**Protect from moisture. Dispense in
tight, light-resistant container (USP).**
Keep this and all drugs out of the
reach of children.
Mfd. by: Novartis Pharmaceuticals Corp.
Suffern, New York 10901
Dist. by: Novartis Pharmaceuticals Corp.
East Hanover, New Jersey 07936
©Novartis

Courtesy of Novartis

NDC 0008-1211-14

Pristiq ®
desvenlafaxine

Extended-Release Tablets

50 mg *

Note: Give attached Medication
Guide when dispensing Pristiq®.

℞ only
Wyeth ®

Unit of Use
14
Tablets

SEALED FOR YOUR PROTECTION
*Each tablet contains 76 mg desvenlafaxine
succinate equivalent to 50 mg desvenlafaxine.
Usual Dosage: See package insert.
Wyeth Pharmaceuticals Inc.
Philadelphia, PA 19101
PAA011337

Store at 20° to 25°C (68° to 77°F); excursions
permitted to 15° to 30°C (59° to 86°F).
[See USP Controlled Room
Temperature]

Package intended to be dispensed
as a unit.

U.S. Patents: See
package insert.   LOT   EXP

Copyright Pfizer Inc. Reproduced with permission.

NDC 0088-1102-47

60 mg   **Hoechst Marion Roussel**

ALLEGRA™
(fexofenadine hydrochloride)

60 mg

100 Capsules

50013685

Each capsule contains: fexofenadine hydrochloride   60 mg
Dosage and Administration: Read package insert for prescribing
information. **CAUTION:** Federal law prohibits dispensing without prescription. **Warning:** Keep out of reach of children. **Pharmacist:** Dispense in tight, light-resistant container as
defined in USP. Important: This package is
not child resistant. Store at controlled room
temperature 68-77°F (20-25°C).

© 1997, Hoechst Marion Roussel, Inc.

US Patents 4,254,129; 5,375,693; 5,578,610

Mfd jointly by:
Hoechst Marion Roussel, Inc.
Kansas City, MO 64137 USA
and
Marion & Company
Manoti, Puerto Rico 00674

Courtesy of Hoechst Marion Roussell, Inc.

NDC 0048-1020-05

Code 3P1025

SYNTHROID ®

**(Levothyroxine Sodium
Tablets, USP)**

25 mcg   (0.025 mg)

1000 TABLETS

Rx only

BASF Pharma   **knoll** ®

See full prescribing
information for dosage
and administration.

Dispense in a tight,
light-resistant
container as described
in USP.

Store at 25°C (77°F);
excursions permitted to
15°-30°C (59°-86°F). [See
USP Controlled Room
Temperature].
**Knoll Pharmaceutical
Company**
Mount Olive, NJ 07828
USA

7897-03

Courtesy of Abbott Laboratories, 2002

**Store at Controlled Room Temperature
20°-25°C (68°-77°F) [see USP].**

Dispense in original, unopened container.

DOSAGE AND USE
See accompanying prescribing information.

Each tablet contains 0.4 mg nitroglycerin.

**Keep this and all drugs out
of the reach of children.**

Warning—To prevent loss of potency, keep
these tablets in the original container or in a
supplemental Nitroglycerin container
specifically labeled as being suitable for
Nitroglycerin Tablets. Close tightly
immediately after each use.

Manufactured by:
Pfizer Pharmaceuticals LLC
Vega Baja, PR 00694   **8212**

NDC 0071-0418-24
Rx only

100 Sublingual Tablets

Nitrostat ®
(Nitroglycerin
Tablets, USP)   0.4

0.4 mg (1/150 gr)

05-5873-32-2

Distributed by
Pfizer **Parke-Davis**
Division of Pfizer Inc, NY, NY 10017

Label is reproduced with permission of Pfizer Inc.

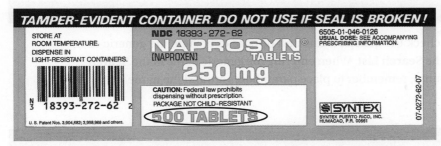

TAMPER-EVIDENT CONTAINER. DO NOT USE IF SEAL IS BROKEN !

STORE AT ROOM TEMPERATURE. DISPENSE IN LIGHT-RESISTANT CONTAINERS.

NDC 18393-272-62

NAPROSYN®
[NAPROXEN] TABLETS
250 mg

CAUTION: Federal law prohibits dispensing without prescription. PACKAGE NOT CHILD-RESISTANT

500 TABLETS

6505-01-046-0126
USUAL DOSE: SEE ACCOMPANYING PRESCRIBING INFORMATION.

SYNTEX
SYNTEX PUERTO RICO, INC. HUMACAO, P.R. 00661

18393-272-62

U.S. Patent Nos. 3,904,682; 3,998,966 and others.

07-0272-62-07

Courtesy of Roche Laboratories Inc.

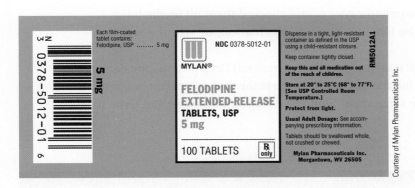

Each film-coated tablet contains: Felodipine, USP .... 5 mg

NDC 0378-5012-01
MYLAN®

FELODIPINE EXTENDED-RELEASE TABLETS, USP
5 mg

100 TABLETS
Rx only

Dispense in a tight, light-resistant container as defined in the USP using a child-resistant closure.

Keep container tightly closed.

Keep this and all medication out of the reach of children.

Store at 20° to 25°C (68° to 77°F). [See USP Controlled Room Temperature.]

Protect from light.

Usual Adult Dosage: See accompanying prescribing information.

Tablets should be swallowed whole, not crushed or chewed.

Mylan Pharmaceuticals Inc. Morgantown, WV 26505

RM5012A1

Courtesy of Mylan Pharmaceuticals Inc.

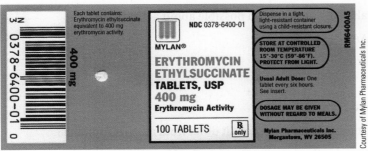

Each tablet contains: Erythromycin ethylsuccinate equivalent to 400 mg erythromycin activity.

NDC 0378-6400-01
MYLAN®

ERYTHROMYCIN ETHYLSUCCINATE TABLETS, USP
400 mg
Erythromycin Activity

100 TABLETS
Rx only

Dispense in a tight, light-resistant container using a child-resistant closure.

STORE AT CONTROLLED ROOM TEMPERATURE 15°-30°C (59°-86°F). PROTECT FROM LIGHT.

Usual Adult Dose: One tablet every six hours. See insert.

DOSAGE MAY BE GIVEN WITHOUT REGARD TO MEALS.

Mylan Pharmaceuticals Inc. Morgantown, WV 26505

RM6400A5

Courtesy of Mylan Pharmaceuticals Inc.

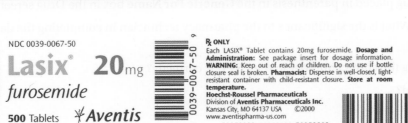

NDC 0039-0067-50

Lasix® 20 mg
furosemide
500 Tablets ✦*Aventis*

Rx ONLY
Each LASIX® Tablet contains 20mg furosemide. **Dosage and Administration:** See package insert for dosage information. **WARNING:** Keep out of reach of children. Do not use if bottle closure seal is broken. **Pharmacist:** Dispense in well-closed, light-resistant container with child-resistant closure. **Store at room temperature.**

Hoechst-Roussel Pharmaceuticals Division of Aventis Pharmaceuticals Inc. Kansas City, MO 64137 USA   ©2000 www.aventispharma-us.com

0039-0067-50

50058803 50058803 **50058803**

Courtesy of Aventis Pharmaceuticals

NDC 0083-0052-30

Tegretol® 100 mg
carbamazepine USP

Chewable Tablets

100 tablets

Rx only

℧ **NOVARTIS**

EXP.   LOT

0083-0052-30

5000098
Dosage: See package insert. Do not store above 30°C (86°F). Protect from light and moisture. Dispense in tight, light-resistant container (USP).

Keep this and all drugs out of the reach of children.

©Novartis

Novartis Pharmaceuticals Corporation East Hanover, New Jersey 07936

Courtesy of Novartis

EXERCISE II

Referring to the labels in Exercise I, check the generic name and be sure to include the generic or brand name for each of the drugs in the **Search List**. When entering the generic name in the **Search List** under the **Generic for Name** column, remember to place parentheses around the name.

EXERCISE III

After you have entered the drugs into the computer system and checked them off on the invoice, they will be stored on the shelf. Check the label for storage information, or visit the website *www.drugs.com/pro*

At the website, you can do a professional search at the FDA Professional Drug Information database. Simply enter the drug you are looking for, and you will be taken to the professional monograph (FDA) for this drug and other drugs in the same class. Find the storage information and write it down, along with the name of the drug.

CRITICAL THINKING

1. Why should the pharmacy technician enter all of the information possible about a drug?

2. What are the differences between AWP and AAC?

3. When would you use the MAC pricing for a drug?

4. What does NDC # mean?

5. Why does the manufacturer have to be entered correctly?

6. When is a UPC code used instead of an NDC number, and how does it differ from an NDC number?

7. Why is the generic name of the drug placed in parenthesis in the **Generic For Name** box in the Drug screen?

8. Why is the sig code default used? What is the significance to the pharmacy technician in completing the daily workload?

9. What is the significance of entering the correct number in the **CS#** box correctly?

10. When is the price quote block used?

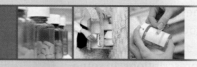

CHAPTER 4

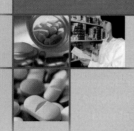

Entering Insurance Claim Information

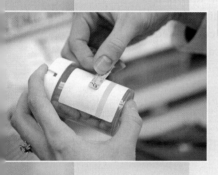

LEARNING OBJECTIVES

1. Describe the responsibilities of an insurance specialist.
2. Point out the significance of a BIN number.
3. Explain the pharmacy ID number.
4. Detail the information needed to process an insurance claim.
5. Explain why a cash fill override might be used instead of processing the insurance claim.
6. Delineate the different types of Rx information needed to process an insurance claim.
7. Discuss the pharmacy information required to complete a claim.
8. Explain workers' compensation and diagnosis codes.
9. Explain the reply process and the importance of prior authorizations.

Setting up and entering insurance claims are tasks that have to be accomplished with every prescription or medical supply order. This chapter looks at the insurance information that must be entered into the various insurance screens containing patient and prescription information needed to process a claim for payment. The many screens involved in processing insurance are necessary for electronically transmitting the claim to the perspective insurance payer. The pharmacist and the pharmacy technician must be able to reply to the insurance payer properly when the claim is rejected for payment.

The pharmacy technician plays an essential role in the insurance claims process, which allows the pharmacist to spend more time with the patient and to address clinical issues. When processing claims, the pharmacy technician is responsible for selecting the physician or provider correctly, and the patient's health insurance information also must be entered accurately.

Pharmacy technicians in some small pharmacies handle the entire computer processes, entering the patient, physician, medication, and insurance information, as well as helping to fill prescriptions. In some large pharmacies, pharmacy technicians handle insurance claims and may be referred to as **insurance specialists**.

The pharmacy, of course, has to be paid for the medication and its services. Therefore, the correct information must be entered and forwarded to the health plan insurance provider.

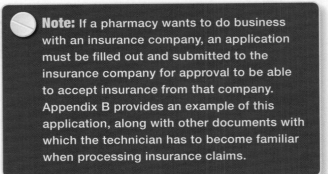

Note: If a pharmacy wants to do business with an insurance company, an application must be filled out and submitted to the insurance company for approval to be able to accept insurance from that company. Appendix B provides an example of this application, along with other documents with which the technician has to become familiar when processing insurance claims.

ENTERING INSURANCE INFORMATION

On the left side of the screen under **Main-1** is a button labeled **Insurance**, which will pop up when you click on it (Figure 4-1). This is the screen you will use to enter information about the different insurance plans and their electronic claims processing information. The pharmacy has contracted with these insurance plans to accept and process electronic claims to pay for the medications and services rendered to patients who have a contract with the same insurance plan.

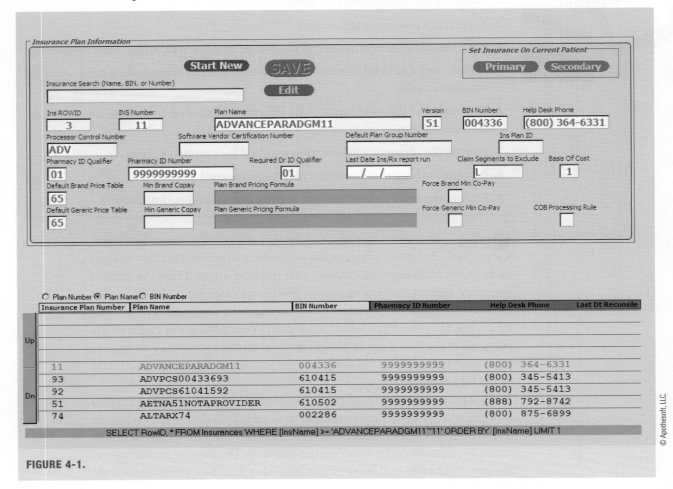

FIGURE 4-1.

© Apothesoft, LLC.

If you are searching for a specific insurance provider, go to **Insurance Search** inside the *Insurance Plan Information* box. Simply type the **Plan Name**, the **BIN Number** (Bank Identification Number), or the **Plan Number**.

To add a new plan to the computer system, click on the **Start New** button at the top of the *Insurance Plan Information* box (Figure 4-3). Most of the information in this box will clear to allow for the new insurance plan information to be entered. The computer will automatically fill in the boxes **Ins ROWID** and **INS Number**. This information indicates the row number of the insurance plan, and the insurance number represents the order in which the insurance plan was added to the list. The numbers will continue to count up in numeric order even if a plan is removed from the list.

> **Note:** The manner in which the insurance is searched for depends on which order the insurance plans are listed in the **Search List** at the bottom of the screen. If the Plan Number is checked, the plans are listed in order (Figure 4-2). If the Plan Name is checked, the plans are listed in alphabetical order. If the BIN Number is checked, the plans are listed in numerical order.

The cursor will advance to the **Plan Name** box. Enter the plan name and hit `ENTER` or `TAB` to advance to the **BIN Number** box. You will notice that the cursor skipped the **Version** box, which contains the number **51,** representing that the *Specifications for NCPDP version 5.1* are

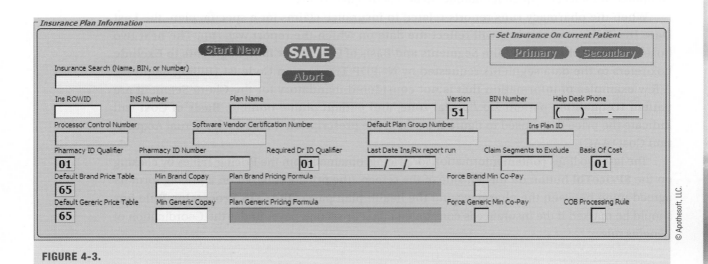

Insurance Plan Number	Plan Name	BIN Number	Pharmacy ID Number	Help Desk Phone	Last Dt Reconsile
11	ADVANCEPARADGM11	004336	9999999999	(800) 364-6331	
93	ADVPCS00433693	610415	9999999999	(800) 345-5413	
92	ADVPCS61041592	610415	9999999999	(800) 345-5413	
51	AETNA51NOTAPROVIDER	610502	9999999999	(888) 792-8742	
74	ALTARX74	002286	9999999999	(800) 875-6899	

SELECT RowID, * FROM Insurances WHERE [InsName] >= 'ADVANCEPARADGM11~11' ORDER BY [InsName] LIMIT 1

© Apothesoft, LLC.

FIGURE 4-2.

FIGURE 4-3.

© Apothesoft, LLC.

being used as a guideline for completing the insurance claims. The individual states will have additional specifications for insurance billing for Medicaid. The state specifications also will be based on NCPDP (National Council for Prescription Drug Programs) standards. NCPDP creates and promotes data interchange standards for the pharmacy services sector of the health care industry.

The **BIN Number** (Bank Identification Number) is a unique number used for routing the pharmacy claim electronically to the proper payer. The number will appear on the patient's insurance card. It also will be provided by the insurance provider when a contract is established between the pharmacy and the insurance provider. The next box, **Help Desk Phone**, provides a number for the pharmacist or the pharmacy technician to call for assistance with processing a claim that may have been rejected, or for other needed assistance. If the Help Desk is busy and if no reject codes are being sent back, someone at the pharmacy should speak personally with someone at the Help Desk to determine the reason for rejecting the claim.

The **Processor Control Number** box refers to the processor that will electronically receive and adjudicate the prescription claim. This processor may be a Pharmacy Benefits Manager (PBM) or the Card Issuer. The **Software Vendor Certification Number** box contains the software number that certifies the ability of the software product and user to submit readable HIPAA-compliant transactions electronically. This certification ensures that claims will be paid. The **Default Plan Group Number** box designates the group plan number for the insurance plan provided to employees through an employer. The **Ins Plan ID** box will contain the identification number for the insurance company that will pay for the pharmacy claim.

The **Pharmacy ID Qualifier** and **Pharmacy ID Number** boxes contain information about the pharmacy. The qualifier ID is a two-digit code to identify the number that is being used to identify the claim submitter. In this case, the **NPI** (National Pharmacy Identification) qualifier is issued by NPPES (National Plan & Provider Enumeration System). To obtain an ID Qualifier and ID Number information, the pharmacy must submit an application to the National Plan & Provider Enumeration System (NPPES), which will issue the National Pharmacy Identification (NPI) qualifier. The NPI is a Health Insurance Portability and Accountability Act (HIPAA) Administration Simplification Standard.

For the information in the **Required Dr ID Qualifier** box, the computer would reference the information from the **Dr-Scrn** *Doctor License Information* box. Depending on the type of payer, the computer will select the qualifier number to be inserted in this box.

When the pharmacy runs reports related to insurance claims for a specific plan, the **Last Date Ins/Rx report run** box will reflect the date on which the report was run. The next two boxes are for exclusion of Claim Segments and Basis of Cost. The **Claim Segments to Exclude** box refers to the data segments requested by NCPDP Transaction Code B1 (Billing Request). A few examples of information that is not considered mandatory for the Claim Segment are patient ID qualifier, patient zip / postal zone, and patient phone number. **Basis of Cost** will indicate the price being used to figure the cost of the prescription—such as the Actual Acquisition Cost (AAC).

The last two lines contain information for pricing, obtained from the Pricing Tables by clicking on the **$PriceTbl** button on the left side of the screen. The pricing is based on a pricing formula agreed upon between the pharmacy and the health plan payer. The **COB Processing Rule** box should be marked if the insurance is considered a first or second payer under the Coordination of Benefits rule.

PROCESSING AN INSURANCE CLAIM

On the lefthand side of the main screen is a button labeled **ClaimXmit** (Figure 4-4). Click on this button to process a claim.

After you click on the **ClaimXmit** button, the screen will change and six different claim buttons will appear, along with three reply buttons (Figure 4-5). Each of these buttons contains information for processing a claim or replying to a payer to provide additional information requested for processing the claim.

Claim-S1 Processing

Once a prescription is filled and saved into the computer system, the **Claim-S1** screen will pop up. The current prescription number will appear in the **Rx#** box at the top of the screen. If the patient had provided insurance information to the pharmacy previously, that information will appear in the screen and the claim can be processed.

After opening the screen for **Claim-S1**, you will see that the screen is divided into three boxes (Figure 4-6), each representing a segment that corresponds to the information required by the *NCPDP Version 5.1 Transactions.*

The first box is ***Claim Segment A - Header*** (Figure 4-7), and the information for this box is pulled from the information that was entered in the ***Insurance Plan Information*** box in **Main-1**. All of this information is mandatory for electronic processing. If the Insurance Information box was completed with all

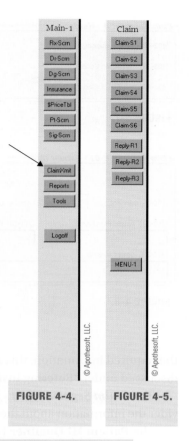

FIGURE 4-4.   **FIGURE 4-5.**

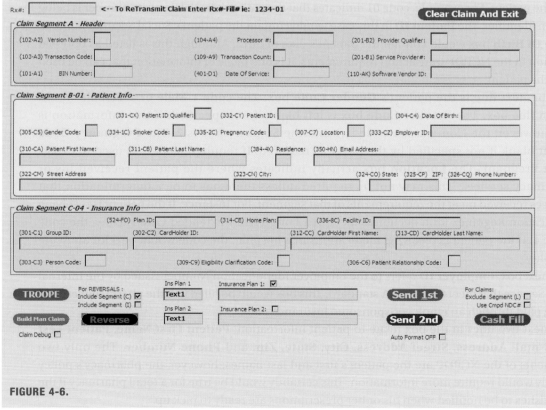

FIGURE 4-6.

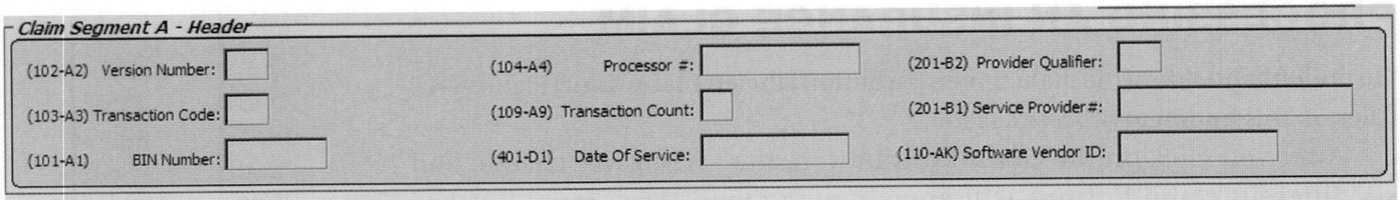

FIGURE 4-7.

Claim Segment A - Header

(102-A2) Version Number: (104-A4) Processor #:   (201-B2) Provider Qualifier:

(103-A3) Transaction Code: (109-A9) Transaction Count: (201-B1) Service Provider #:

(101-A1) BIN Number: (401-D1) Date Of Service: (110-AK) Software Vendor ID:

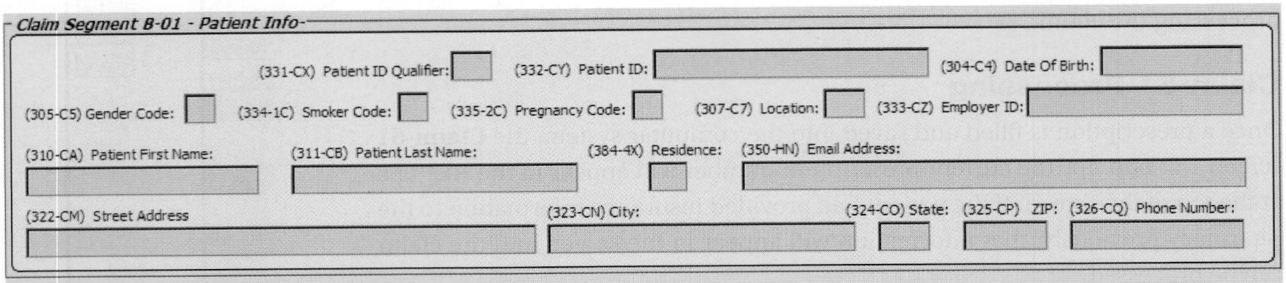

© Apothesoft, LLC.

FIGURE 4-8.

Claim Segment B-01 - Patient Info

(331-CX) Patient ID Qualifier: (332-CY) Patient ID: (304-C4) Date Of Birth:

(305-C5) Gender Code: (334-1C) Smoker Code: (335-2C) Pregnancy Code: (307-C7) Location: (333-CZ) Employer ID:

(310-CA) Patient First Name: (311-CB) Patient Last Name: (384-4X) Residence: (350-HN) Email Address:

(322-CM) Street Address   (323-CN) City: (324-CO) State: (325-CP) ZIP: (326-CQ) Phone Number:

© Apothesoft, LLC.

the required information, this box should not have to be filled out. (Refer back to the information discussed under "Entering Insurance Information" to review each box and what it represents.)

The **Claim Segment B-01 - Patient Info** (Figure 4-8) box is used to provide the health plan provider the information about the subscriber to the health plan.

The **Patient ID Qualifier** box designates the type of identification information being used to identify the patient. For example, code 01 indicates that the patient's Social Security number is being used as an identifier. The **Patient ID** in this case would contain the patient's Social Security number. The **Date Of Birth** box would contain the patient's date of birth. Although this is listed as optional information in the NCPDP transaction requirements, it is one piece of information that can be used to verify the patient.

On the next line is the patient's **Gender Code** box. The code 1-Male or 2-Female would appear in this box. The **Smoker Code** box is left blank if not specified. If this information is known, however, the Non-smoker code is 1 and the Smoker code is 2. The **Pregnancy Code** box is left blank if not specified by the payer as required. If required, code 1 is used to designate Not Pregnant. The **Location** box actually indicates where the patient received his or her pharmacy services. This may not be required unless there has to be a determination that the services received meet the requirements of that segment. For instance, if the patient is receiving the medication Regranex for a decubitus ulcer in a Long Term / Extended Care Facility, the code would be 4. If the patient is receiving medications in a hospital, the code would be 9 for an Acute Care Facility.

The next box, **Employer ID** refers to the Employer Identification Number issued by the Internal Revenue Service that meets the HIPAA standard. This box would be filled in if the pharmacy services are being paid through an employer-sponsored insurance plan.

The next two lines in the box relate to patient information: **Patient First Name**, **Patient Last Name**, **E-mail Address**, **Street Address**, **City**, **State**, **Zip**, and **Phone Number**. The only two requirements of the NCPDP are the patient's first and last names; however, the pharmacy's policy most likely would require more information. This certainly would be true for a retail pharmacy if the patient wishes to be notified when his or her prescriptions are ready to pick up.

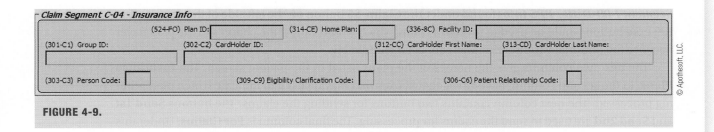

FIGURE 4-9.

The last segment, ***Claim Segment C-04 - Insurance Info*** (Figure 4-9), contains information for processing the insurance claim. The first box on the first line, **Plan ID**, identifies the insurance plan. The **Home Plan** is not required by NCPDP version 5.1. Because the versions of the NCPDP transaction may change from time to time, some information boxes may not have to be filled in. That information, however, could change with future versions and, therefore, the individual boxes are retained in the program fields. The **Facility ID** is filled in only if the **Location** box in the ***Claim Segment B-01*** contains a code other than 1 for Home. For example, if the location Code is for long-term / extended-care facility 4, that facility's ID number would be entered in this box. The facility's ID is its NPI number.

The boxes in the middle line pertain specifically to the insurance plan IDs for the insurance card holder. The **Group ID** would be found on the insurance card along with the **Cardholder ID** and the **Cardholder First Name** and **Cardholder Last Name**. On the last line is the **Person Code** box, which would be filled in with the code 000 or Blank if not specified, or with 001 to indicate that the insurance claim is for the cardholder; this depends on the requirements of the insurance payer.

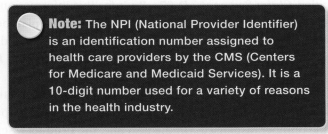

Note: The NPI (National Provider Identifier) is an identification number assigned to health care providers by the CMS (Centers for Medicare and Medicaid Services). It is a 10-digit number used for a variety of reasons in the health industry.

The next box, the **Eligibility Clarification Code**, is used to indicate the pharmacy clarification request. Examples of the values used are as follows: 3 for Full-Time Student, 4 for Disabled Dependent, and 5 for Dependent Parent.

The final box, **Patient Relationship Code**, indicates the relationship of the patient to the cardholder. For example, if the cardholder is the person for whom the claim is being processed, the code 1 would be entered.

Function Buttons for Processing

Across the bottom of the **Claim-S1** screen are several buttons and boxes related to the final processing of the initial claim (refer back to Figure 4-6) before the **Claim-S2** button - Rx Information. On the bottom left, the first button, **TROOPE**, allows for checking on billing information for Medicare Part D, such as online eligibility through the enrollment system known as TROOPE Facilitator. This would be used for an individual who has no proof of enrollment in Medicare Part D.

Once the information is processed through **TROOPE**, the patient's plan will verify that the patient is or is not covered, by way of a computer message. Below the **TROOPE** button is the button **Build Man Claim**, which allows the pharmacist or pharmacy technician to build a claim manually. This would be necessary if the information from the patient screen is not correct or if a new insurance policy had not been added to the system for that patient. Below the **Build Man Claim** button is the checkbox **Claim Debug**, which can be used to debug a claim being processed.

The next column provides for processing **Reversals**. Above the **Reverse** button are two checkboxes that allow for inclusion of information from the ***Claim Segment C-04 - Insurance Info*** and

Segment I-09-DUR / PPS Info (found under the **Claim-S5** button on the left side of the screen). The **Reverse** button would be used to reverse a claim, which would cancel the charges to the plan payer because the pharmacy transaction was cancelled completely.

The next two columns give the names of the plans listed in the patient screen. The **Insurance Plans**, in the second column, have small checkboxes that may be used to indicate which plan is being processed. The next column contains two buttons for sending the claims. The buttons **Send 1st** and **Send 2nd** are used to send the claims for processing. The final column is **For Claims**. Under this column the boxes may be checked to **Exclude Segment - L-10–Compound Info,** found under button **Claim-S4** on the left side of the screen, or **Use Cmpnd NDC** # for processing the insurance claim based on the compound NDC number and ingredients.

The final button, **Cash Fill**, would be used to force a cash sell and override the insurance claim. At times patients want to pay cash instead of using their insurance because, for example, the cash price may be less than the copay for the insurance.

Claim-S2 Button - Rx Information

After completing or checking the information in the fields in the **Claim-S1** screen, you may have to check the information in the **Claim-S2** screen (Figure 4-10). This screen contains one box titled *Claim Segment - D-07 - Rx Info*. This information comes from the **Rx-Scrn** button screen (Figure 4-11). The current Rx # and the insurance plan being used to process the claim appear in boxes above the Segment box. The information generated while filling a prescription or processing a refill prescription will be entered into *Claim Segment - D - 07 Rx Info* box. If a mistake was made while filling the prescription, the claim would be denied.

The first line of boxes in this segment contains information on the type of billing: **Rx / Service Ref # Qualifier** - 01 for Rx billing, **Rx / Service Ref #** = prescription number, and **Quantity Dispensed** = the number dispensed. On the next line, the **Product / Service Qualifier** indicates the type of code

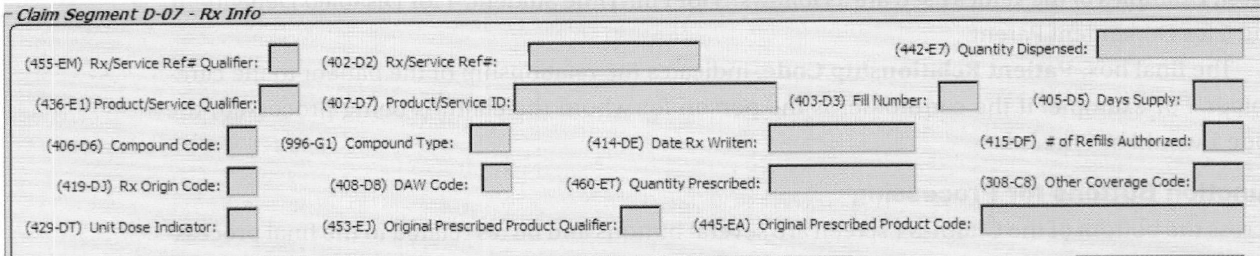

FIGURE 4-10.

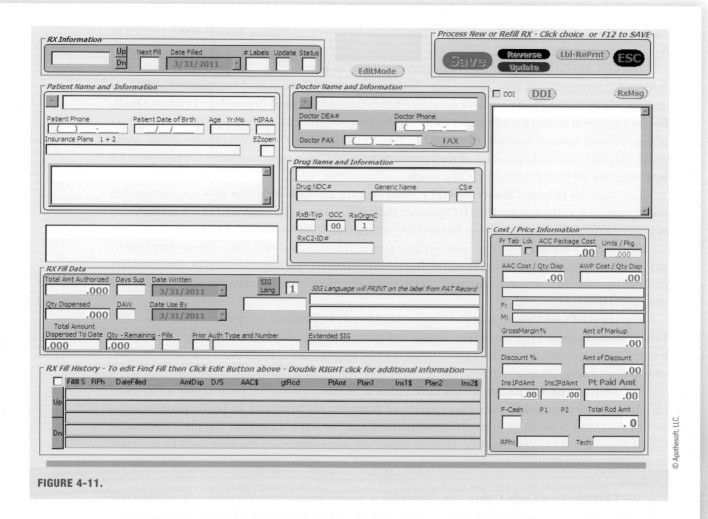

FIGURE 4-11.

© Apothesoft, LLC.

being submitted. For example, if code 03 appears in the box, it indicates that the National Drug Code (NDC) number is being used. Code 00 would be used if a compound is being billed. The **Product / Service ID** box would contain the NDC number. The next two boxes are for the **Fill Number**, which indicates if this is the original prescription—Code 00—or the refill number—Code 1-99—for the prescription being dispensed. The last box in this line, **Days Supply**, indicates the number of days the prescription will last.

The third line of boxes contains the **Compound Code** which contains the code to indicate whether the prescription is a compound. If the prescription is a compound, a 2 would appear in the box. If it is not a compound, either a 0 for Not Specified or a 1 for Not a Compound would appear in the box. The next box contains the **DAW Code** to indicate if the prescriber's instructions were followed regarding generic substitution. For example, if **substitution allowed** pharmacist selected, Code—4 will appear; however, if **substitution not allowed brand drug mandatory by law**, Code—7 will appear.

The next box, **Date Rx Written**, must contain a date that is not greater than the current date and must appear in the following format: CCYYMMDD—example 20101104. The last box, **# of Refills Authorized**, indicates the number of refills for which the prescriber wrote the original prescription. This information is optional under NCPDP version 5.1.

On the fourth line, the box **Rx Origin Code**, indicates how the prescription was initiated. Examples of the codes are as follows: 1-Written, 2-Telephone, 3-Electronic, and 4-Facsimile. The **Quantity Prescribed** code must be 1 or greater. The **Other Coverage Code** box would contain information on whether the patient has other coverage. Those codes represent everything from 0-Not specified to 8 -Claim is billing for copay.

The fifth line of boxes contains information related to unit dosing. The **Unit Dose Indicator** indicates the type of unit dose dispensing. For instance, code-2 indicates Manufacturer unit dose and code-3 indicates Pharmacy unit dose. The boxes labeled **Original Prescribed Product Qualifier** and **Original Prescribed Product Code** are considered optional information under version 5.1 of the National Council for Prescription Drug Programs (NCPDP) *Transaction Codes Guide*. These codes may be found in Appendix K of the *Transaction Codes Guide*, which includes the complete 5.1 version of the NCPDP *Transaction Code Guide*.

The boxes for **Original Prescribed QTY**, **Alternate ID**, and **Scheduled Rx ID #** are not required under version 5.1. The box for **Unit Of Measure** indicates the measurement unit of the prescription being dispensed. These codes are as follows: EA—Each, GM—Grams, and ML Milliliters.

The next two boxes are for intermediary processing. If authorized with code-1 in the **Intermediary Authoriztn ID Type** box, the **Intermediary Authoriztn ID** box must be filled in. Intermediary processing refers to a separate company that handles the processing between the point of sale and the payer company.

The **Level Of Service** box would be required to identify Emergency Service with the code-3. The **Prior Authorization Type Code** box indicates that the **Prior Authorization Number Submitted** box is completed with the number given to allow prior authorization. Eight different codes are possible for prior authorization. An example is medical certification-2.

The **Dispensing Status** box would have either a "P" for a partial fill or a "C" for a complete fill. The **Quantity Intended to be Dispensed** and **Days Supply Intended To Be Dispensed** boxes would show the amount of medication dispensed and the days supply for the prescription for which the claim is being submitted. If these boxes are not completed, the claim will be rejected. The next two lines of boxes are optional under version 5.1; however, they may be required in future versions.

The **Clarification Code Count** box allows for a maximum of three occurrences, so the code would be 1 to 3. The **Clarification Codes** boxes indicate how the pharmacist is clarifying the information. For example, code 3 indicates that the fill is a vacation supply, or 6 for Starter Dose. The pharmacist may enter up to three clarifications.

As you see by looking at all of the information that may be required to process a prescription, there is a lot of opportunity for error. A couple of errors that occur most often are the **DAW** and the **Days Supply Codes**. If the information is incorrect here, the claim will be denied.

Claim-S3 Button - Pharmacy Information, Prescriber Information, and Other Payer Groups

The button **Claim-S3** at the top of the screen contains the current **Rx#** box and which of the two insurance plans is being processed. The *Claim Segment E-02 Pharmacy Info* box contains the **Provider ID Qualifier** box and the **Pharmacy Provider ID** box (Figure 4-12). This information is pulled from the computer system Tools configuration screen for the pharmacy. This information also would appear in the **Claim Segment A–Header** under the **Claim-S1** screen.

The **Claim Segment F-03–Prescriber Info** box contains information about the prescriber. This information would be pulled by the computer from the **Dr-Scrn** button, which indicates the prescriber by **Qualifier**, **Location Code**, **Prescriber Last Name**, and **Prescriber ID**. This box also contains boxes for information pertaining to the **Qualifier**, **Location Code**, **PrimaryCare Provider Last Name**, and **PrimaryCare Provider ID**. This information is required when a primary care prescriber is required by the payer plan.

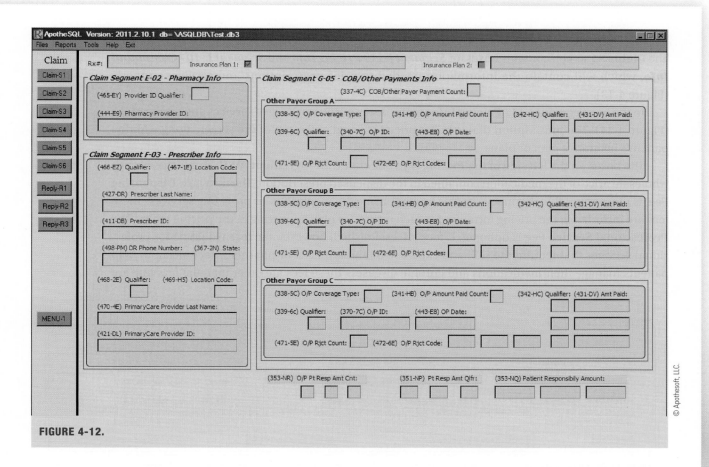

FIGURE 4-12.

The **Claim *Segment G-05–COB/Other Payment Info*** portion of the **Claim-S3** screen provides information about coordinating benefits with other payers. In the top box, ***COB/Other Payor Payment Count***, codes 1 through 3 would appear, representing the number of other payers being processed for the same claim. The number of other payers cannot exceed three. The information for each payer would be pulled from the other payer's insurance information under the **Pt-Scrn** button under **Main-1**.

In the **Other Payor Group A, B, and C** boxes, the information about the other payer is entered. The **O/P Coverage Type** will contain one of the following: Code 01- Primary, 02- Secondary, or 03-Tertiary. No more than three occurrences of other payers are allowed. The count for the **O/P Amount Paid Count** box would indicate the number of occurrences of payment by the other payer, designated by a number from 1 to 3. On the next line, the **Qualifier** box would contain Code -99, indicating that the other's payer identification code is invalid.

The **O/P ID** box would contain the identification number for the payer, and the **O/P Date** box would contain the date on which the other payer's adjudication was determined to be invalid. To the far right are three boxes for **Qualifier** codes, which indicate what the other payers paid for. Examples of these codes are as follows: 02-Shipping, 07-Drug Benefit, and 98-Coupon. The amounts paid will appear in the boxes next to the **Qualifier code** under the **Amt Paid** heading.

The last line in the **Other Payor Group** box contains the **O/P Rjct Count**, which indicates the number of rejections of the other payers, and it must match the number of other payer occurrences. The **O/P Rjct Codes** can be found in the *NCPDP Data Dictionary*, found in Appendix F of the *NCPDP Data Dictionary*. Across the bottom are three boxes each for **O/P Pt Resp Amt Cnt**, **Pt Resp Amt Qlfr**, and **Patient Responsibility Amount**. These boxes have been added under a new *NCPDP version D.0 Claiming Billing* and would be used if required by payer.

Claim-S4 Button - Pricing Information and Compound Information

The **Claim-S4** screen contains boxes for *Segment J-11 - Pricing Info* and *Segment L-10 - Compound Info*, which will contain the information needed to price prescriptions and services properly (Figure 4-13).

In the box *Segment J-11 - Pricing Info* are the boxes to enter pricing of services and medications (Figure 4-14). The prescription that is being priced is listed at the top of the screen along with the patient's insurance plan or plans.

The boxes on the left side of the *Pricing Info* box start with **Ingredient AWP**. This is the average wholesale price of the medication contained in the dispensed prescription. The next box, **Dispensing Fee**, is the amount the pharmacy charges for dispensing the medication or providing services. These fees are included in the pricing formulas for each insurance plan appearing in the pricing tables. The **Professional Service Fee** is optional. If fees are established, however, the fees would be for professional services that require the skill and expertise of a pharmacist or pharmacy technician to help patients manage their medications and chronic diseases. These fees are other than the fees that are

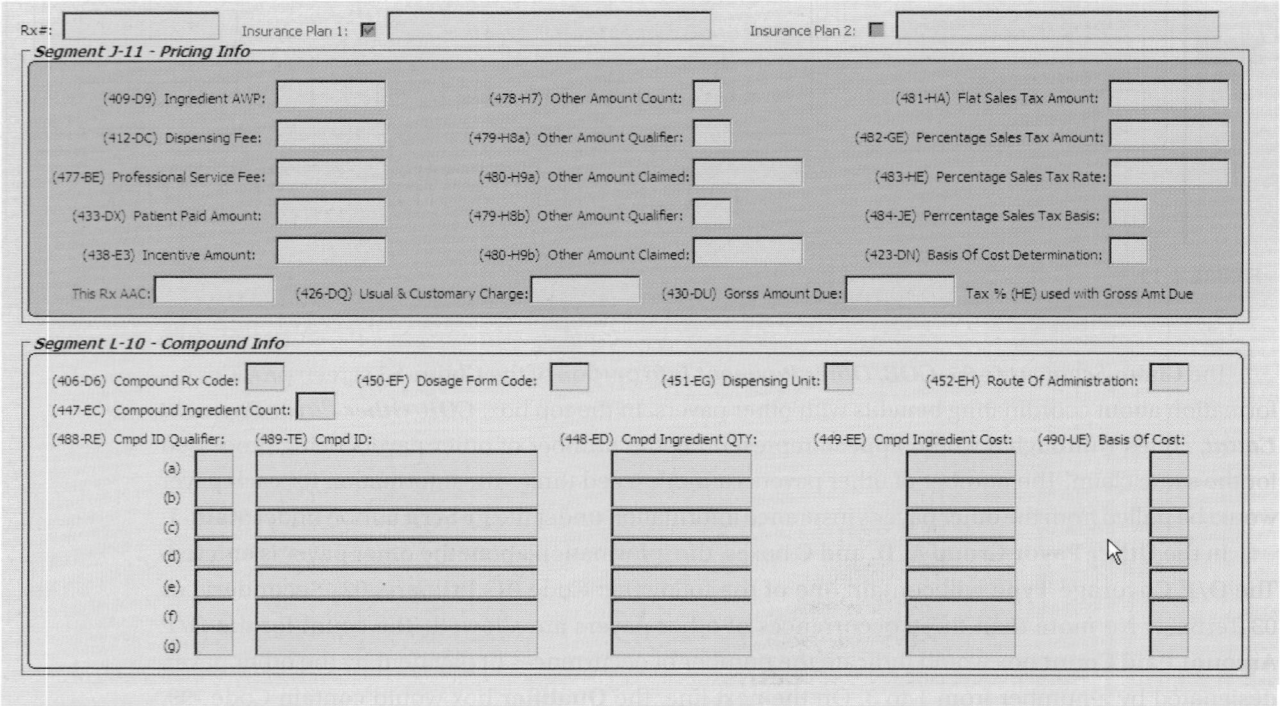

FIGURE 4-13.

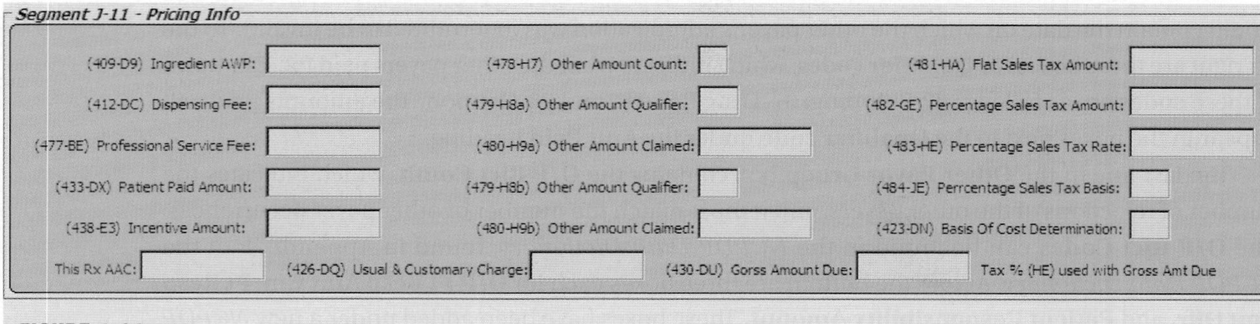

FIGURE 4-14.

© Apothesoft, LLC.

considered Usual and Customary charges for dispensing a medication. The **Patient Paid Amount** is the cost of the dispensed medication to the patient. The last box in this column, **Incentive Amount**, represents a fee submitted by the pharmacy for contractually agreed upon services with the insurance plan. This amount will be included in the **Gross Amount Due**.

The middle column of boxes contains information on the number of occurrences from other claims. The box **Other Amount Count** indicates the number of times another claim has been submitted. The maximum number is 3.

The next box, **Other Amount Qualifier**, identifies the additional incurred cost for this occurrence. Examples of additional costs would be indicated by codes such as 01- Delivery Cost, 02-Shipping Cost, and 03-Postage Cost. The box **Other Amount Claimed** contains the actual dollar amount of the claim. An additional set of boxes is given for another **Amount Qualifier** and **Claim**, allowing for an additional claim for expenses.

The last column of boxes contains additional boxes for completing the pricing of the prescription dispensed or the services of the pharmacist or pharmacy technician. The **Flat Sales Tax Amount** is the amount of sales that would be subject to a tax, if a sales tax is allowed on pharmacy prescriptions and services within the state where the pharmacy is located. The **Percentage Sales Tax Amount** box would be the amount of tax charged. The next box would contain the **Percentage Sales Tax Rate** used to calculate the amount of sales tax. The final two boxes in this column indicate **Percentage Sales Tax Basis** and **Basis Of Cost Determination**. The **Percentage Sales Tax Basis** would be indicated by a code such as 01-Gross Amount Due, 02-Ingredient Cost, or 03-Ingredient Cost + Dispensing. The **Basis of Cost Determination** represents the method by which the ingredient cost is determined. Examples of codes that may be used are as follows: 02-Local Wholesaler, 06-Maximum Allowable Cost, or 07-Usual and Customary.

The bottom line of boxes in the Pricing Info box are the **Rx AAC** (Actual Acquisition Cost) for the prescription being priced, and the **Usual & Customary Charge** for the cash amount charged to the patient for the prescription, exclusive of sales tax and other amounts claimed. Finally, the **Gross Amount Due** indicates the total price claimed for all sources.

The *Segment L-10 - Compound Info* box is used to price the charge for a compound (Figure 4-15). The **Compound Rx Code** box indicates that a compound is being billed when code 2 is entered in the box. The next box, **Dosage Form Code**, indicates the form in which the compound is being dispensed. For instance, if the compound is a suppository, code 04 would appear in the box. The **Dispensing Unit** indicates the unit of measure for the compound, such as Code 1-Each, 2-Grams, or 3-Milliliters. The last box in the top row, **Route Of Administration**, would contain a code indicating the form in which the compounded medication or product is to be taken or used. For example, this might be represented by Code 1-Oral or Code 13-Otic.

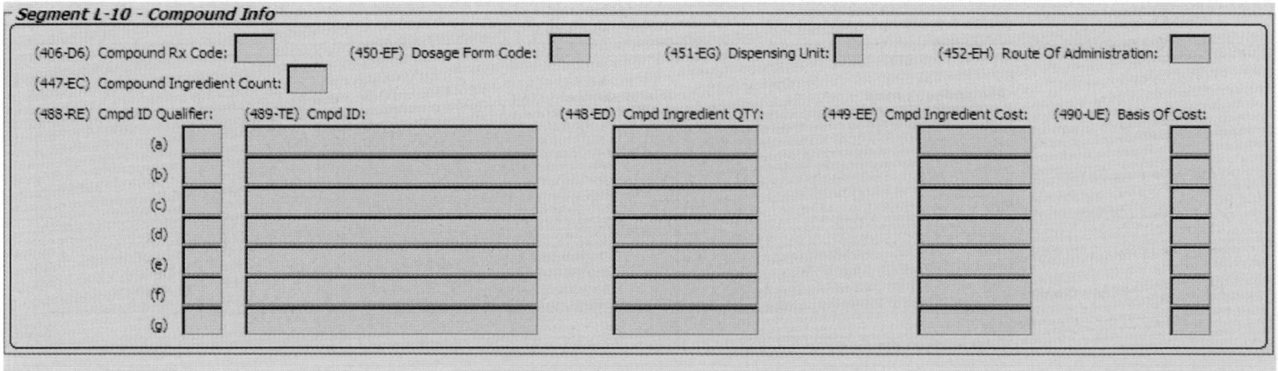

FIGURE 4-15.

The **Compound Ingredient Count** indicates the number of ingredients in the compound. The maximum number of 25 ingredients will be accepted for processing. In the **Cmpd ID Qualifier** column, **code 03** is entered to indicate that the NDC # is being used as the **Cmpd ID** for the ingredient in the next column.

The next two columns, **Cmpd Ingredient QTY** and **Cmpd Ingredient Cost**, simply list the amount of ingredient used and how much that ingredient cost. The last column, **Basis Of Cost**, indicates the method of calculating the drug cost of the ingredient used in the compound. This would be represented by a code such as 01-AWP or 07-Usual & Customary.

Claim-S5 Button - DUR/PPS Information and Prior Authorization Information

At the top of the **Claim-S5** screen appears the prescription that is being processed and the associated insurances (Figure 4-16). The first box for *Segment I-08 - DUR/PPS Info* is used to provide information on the reasons for a Drug Utilization Review or for Professional Pharmacy Services charges (Figure 4-17). The boxes for each group represent the occurrences of charges.

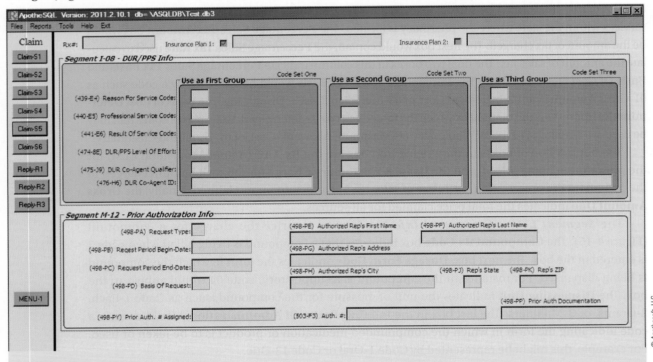

FIGURE 4-16.

FIGURE 4-17.

© Apothesoft, LLC.

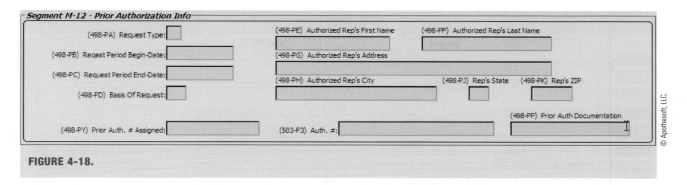

FIGURE 4-18.

The **Reason For Service Code** box indicates why there is a charge, such as the Code DD representing Drug Drug Interaction. Pharmacists provide their professional services to intervene when a conflict in patient therapy arises. When these professional services are rendered, they are coded in the **Professional Service Code** box. The codes representing the type of intervention are two letters such as the following: AS-Patient Assessment, CC-Coordination of Care, DE-Dosing Evaluation/ Determination, and FE- Formulary Enforcement.

The next box provides information indicating the result of the action taken by the pharmacist or the result of the pharmacist's professional services. Some of the codes that would be used in the **Result Of Service Code** box are as follows: 1A-Filled As Is, False Positive, 1C-Filled With Different Dose, or 1D-Filled With Different Directions.

DUR/PPS Level Of Effort indicates the level of effort determined by the complexity of the decision-making or resources utilized by the pharmacist to perform professional services. The codes that would be used here range from 1-Level 1 (lowest) to 15-Level 5 (highest) amount of complexity. The final two lines contain the information for the **DUR Co-Agent Qualifier** and **DUR Co-Agent ID**. The code for the co-existing agent contributing to the DUR event is indicated by the Qualifier 03, and the ID would be the Co-Agent NDC number.

The next box is the screen **Segment M-12 - Prior Authorization Info** (Figure 4-18). The **Request Type** box indicates what type of prior authorization request is being submitted. The request codes for the types of request are as follows: 1-Initial, 2-Recertification, and 3- Revised. Directly below the type of request are the **Request Period Begin-Date** and the **Request Period End-Date** boxes. The begin date represents the initial date of the claim, and the end date denotes the date of recertification. The **Basis Of Request** box would contain the **Code PR** if the plan requires the prior authorization. The boxes to the right are designated for the authorized representative's (the ordering physician) information.

Across the bottom of this box are the boxes for **Prior Auth # Assigned, Auth. #,** and **Prior Auth Documentation**. The authorization numbers are assigned for tracking and the type of information to support the prior authorization.

Claim-S6 Button - Worker's Compensation Information, Clinical Information, and Coupon Information

The last button on the left side of the screen for insurance claim processing is **Claim-S6** (Figure 4-19). Again, at the top of the screen, the current prescription number appears along with the insurance plans for that patient.

The *Segment H-06 - Worker's Compensation Info* box contains those code elements needed for submission of a Workmen's Compensation claim (Figure 4-20). These claims are paid when an employee was injured or became ill while on the job. The employee is covered either by a state

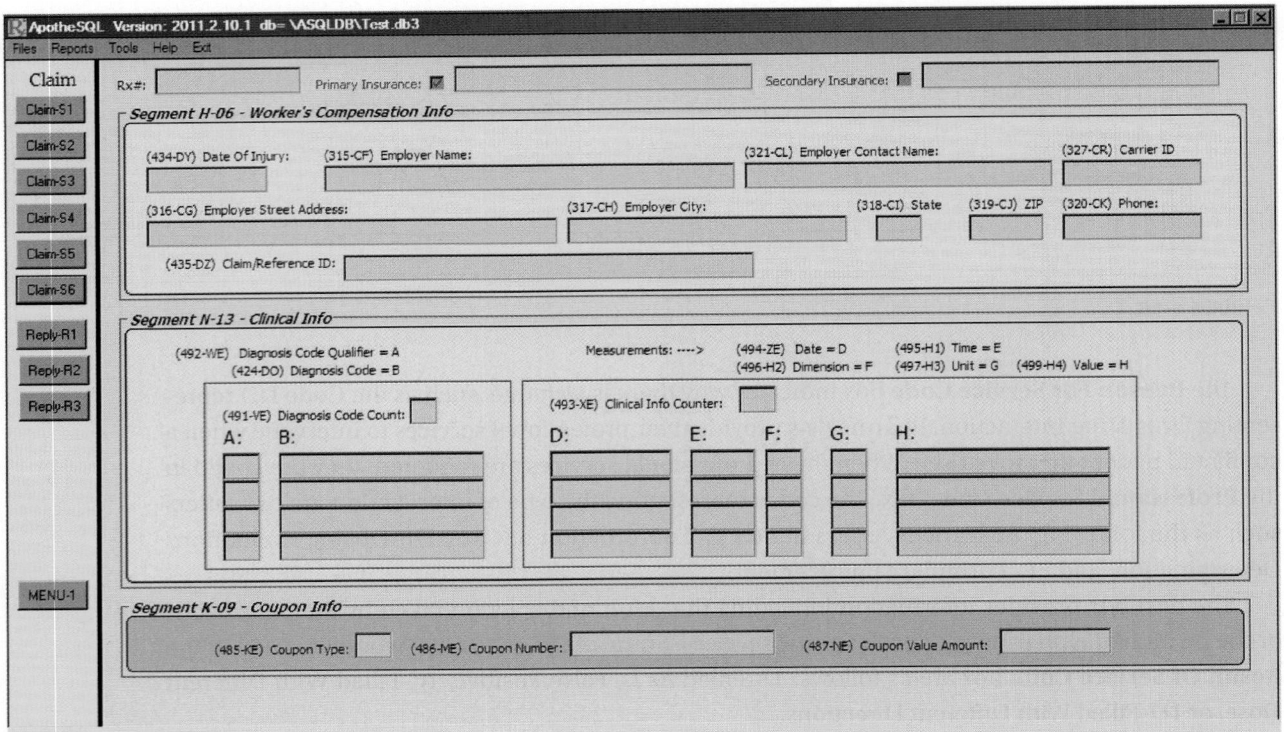

© Apothesoft, LLC.

FIGURE 4-19.

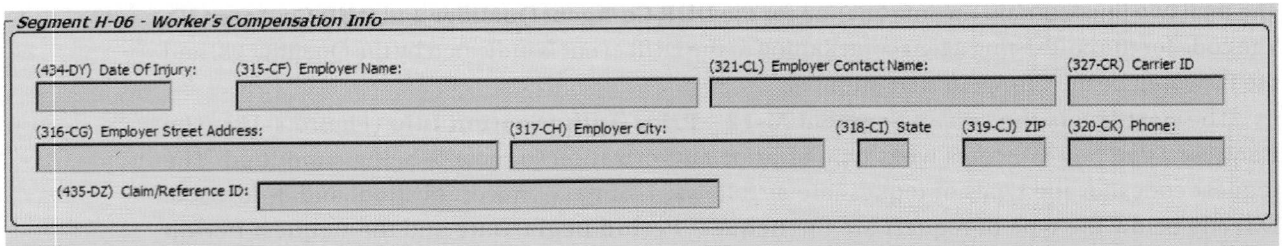

© Apothesoft, LLC.

FIGURE 4-20.

plan or a federal plan, depending on the Workmen's Compensation insurance carried by his or her employer. The pharmacist or pharmacy technician will have to contact the patient's employer to verify eligibility for Workmen's Compensation and to find out the insurance carrier and the carrier's ID number. The date of injury also should be verified.

Most of the information in this segment is optional except when a COB (coordination of benefits) claim is being processed. The **Date Of Injury** box information is mandatory and must be submitted in the CCYYMMDD format. The **Carrier ID** box information is required for a Coordination of Benefits claim, along with the **Claim /Reference ID** box. After pharmacy technicians have received the information from the employer, they may have to contact the insurance company directly to find out exactly what information is needed.

The ***Segment N-13 - Clinical Info*** box contains the information pertaining to the patient diagnosis (Figure 4-21). The index at the top of the box indicates what type of information is to be included in boxes A through H. The **Diagnosis Code Qualifier - A** is 01, indicating that ICD9

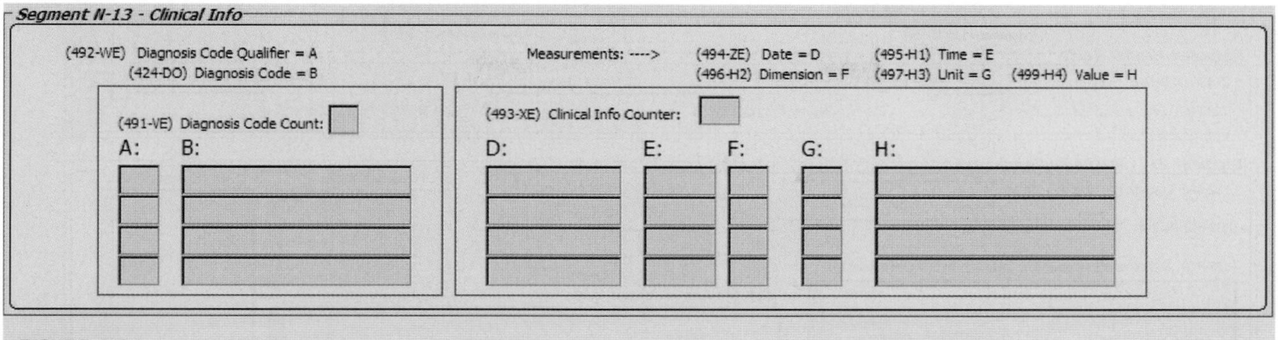

Segment N-13 - Clinical Info

(492-WE) Diagnosis Code Qualifier = A Measurements: ----> (494-ZE) Date = D (495-H1) Time = E
(424-DO) Diagnosis Code = B (496-H2) Dimension = F (497-H3) Unit = G (499-H4) Value = H

(491-VE) Diagnosis Code Count: [ ] (493-XE) Clinical Info Counter: [ ]

A: B: D: E: F: G: H:

FIGURE 4-21.

codes are to be used. The **Diagnosis Code - B** is the appropriate ICD9 code for the diagnosis. The **Date - D** is the date the information was collected, written in the CCYYMMDD format. **Time - E** is the time the information was collected and is to be entered in the 24-hour format HHMM. The **Dimension - F** indicates the clinical domain using codes such as 01-Blood Pressure, 03-Temperature, 08- Calcium, 14-Weight, 16-Height, and 99-Other.

Unit - G is indicated by 01 for inches and 03 for pounds. **Value - H** denotes the actual inches or pounds. The last two boxes, **Diagnosis Code Count** and **Clinical Info Counter**, call for a number 1 through 5 to indicate the number of occurrences.

The final *Segment K-09 - Coupon Info* box contains information about any coupon used by the patient at the pharmacy (Figure 4-22). The **Coupon Type** box indicates the type of coupon using the codes: 01-Price discount, 02- Free product, and 99- Other. The **Coupon Number** box contains the number on the coupon, and the **Coupon Value Amount** is the face value of the coupon presented.

Note: In applying for Workmen's Compensation, the insurance company may provide a list of drugs it will cover or a third party insurance card may be issued to the claimant. If the drugs that are being provided through the list or third party do not meet the claimant's needs, the pharmacist may have to contact the insurance company directly.

Note: A pharmacy technician who is trained to handle insurance claims is valuable to the operation of the pharmacy. The process of handling insurance is automatized with the use of sophisticated pharmacy programs, but when a problem arises that is out of the ordinary, the pharmacist and the pharmacy technician have to know how to handle that problem.

Reply-R1 Button - Header Reply, Status Reply, and Claim Reply

After the pharmacy has submitted a claim to the patient's insurance provider, the provider will respond if the claim poses any problems. At the top of each of the screens for the **Reply** buttons are the prescription number and the insurance information the response is referencing.

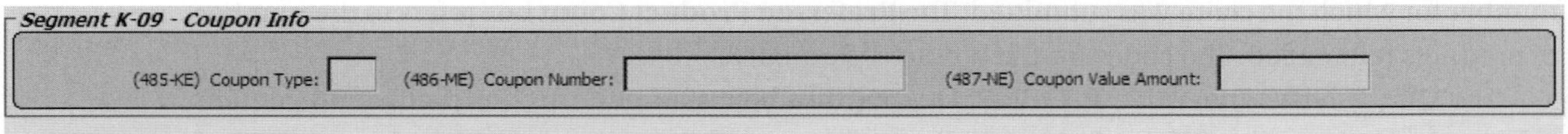

Segment K-09 - Coupon Info

(485-KE) Coupon Type: [ ] (486-ME) Coupon Number: [ ] (487-NE) Coupon Value Amount: [ ]

FIGURE 4-22.

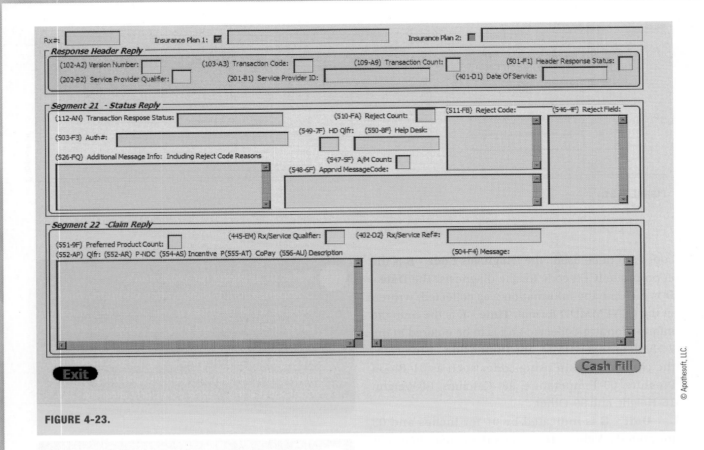

FIGURE 4-23.

© Apothesoft, LLC.

At the top of the **Reply-R1** button is the *Response Header Reply* box, which contains the same information that was provided to the insurance payer in the **Claim Segment A - Header** found under the **Claim-S1** button (Figure 4-23). The only different information is the **Header Response Status** box, which will contain the code A, for Accepted.

The *Segment 21 - Status Reply* block will contain information pertaining to the claim and why or if the claim is rejected. The **Transaction Response Status** box would contain either the code P- Paid or D- Duplicate of Paid. The **Reject Count** may not exceed 5. The **Reject Code** and the **Reject Field** boxes are used to list the rejection codes and reasons for rejecting the claim. The **Auth#** box would contain an assigned code of up to 20 digits in length and is required to identify the transaction. The **HD QLFR** (Help Desk Qualifier) would be a code 01 or whatever code is provided by payer. The **Help Desk** box would contain the telephone number for the help desk. The **Additional Message Info** box is used for free-form text to allow for a message and also **Including Reject Code Reasons**. The **A/M Count** box would contain the number of responses appearing in the **Apprvd Message Code** box. These codes are as follows: 001-Generic Available, 002- Non-formulary Drug, and 003- Maintenance Drug.

The *Segment 22 - Claim Reply* box contains information related to the claim. The **Rx/Service Qualifier** box code is 1, for Rx Billing. The box for the **Rx/Service Ref #** will contain the prescription number for which the claim was submitted. The **Preferred Product Count** box refers to the number of products referenced. The codes for the box are 1 through 3.

The **Qlfr, P-NDC, Incentive P, CoPay, Description** box is a free-form box that would contain information such as the **Qlfr** code 03 to indicate that the NDC number is being referenced. Also,

P-NDC refers to the Preferred Product ID, which denotes the product's NDC numbers. In addition, **Incentive P**, **CoPay**, and **Description** information from the insurance plan payer will appear in the box. This information refers to Preferred Product Incentive, Preferred Provider Incentive, and Preferred Product Description. Preferred products are those that the insurance plan prefers and are represented by the amount of copay, which is determined by the established tier of the insurance payer. The tier is a listing of preferred medications with the lowest cost drugs, usually generics, having the lowest copay amount. The **Message** box allows for free-form text to provide an explanation for the preferred product or any other information pertaining to the claim.

The bottom of the screen has two buttons. One is used to **Exit** the screen after looking over the information from the insurance provider, and the other to change from an insurance claim to a **Cash Fill**.

Reply - R2 Button - Price Payment Information and Insurance Information

Again at the top of the screen, the prescription number and insurance plan information appears referencing the prescription to which the response information is related (Figure 4-24).

The **Segment 23 - Price Payment Info** box contains the information on how the prescription was priced. It also indicates the **Net Pharmacy Profit**. Much of this segment is considered optional under the guidelines of version 5.1. The only information required is the information that was used to arrive at a final reimbursement. All information may be reported back, however, if it was used in processing the claim.

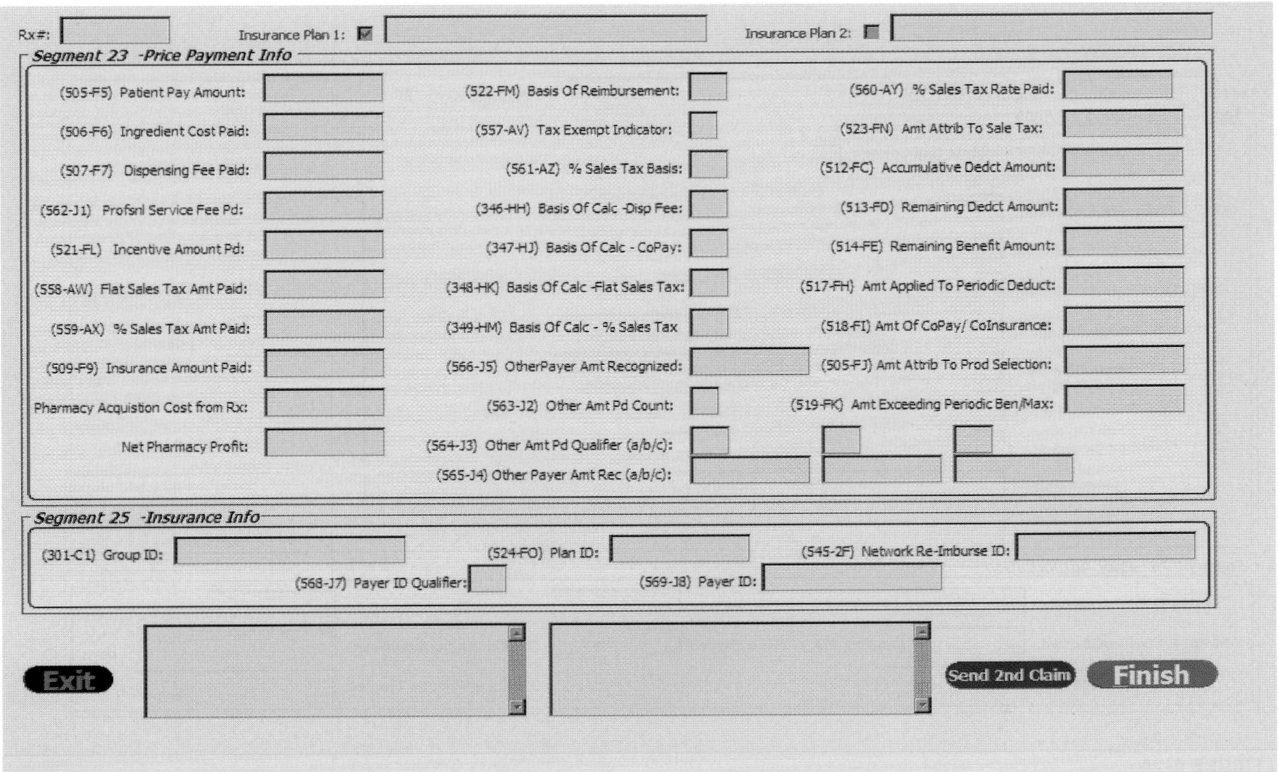

FIGURE 4-24.

The *Segment 25 - Insurance Info* box contains the boxes to enter insurance information. These boxes would be completed in the response when the card holder or the employer group has to be identified. Under the guidelines of version 5.1, this information would be completed by the responding insurance payer, depending on the situation or requirement.

At the bottom of the screen, one button is used to **Exit** the screen and review. The other two buttons are used to indicate that the information is being sent back to the responder, **Send 2nd Claim**, as a second claim, or to respond, **Finish**, the claim is complete. Two additional boxes may be used to enter free text that explains any of the responses to the claim for further information about the response to the claim.

Reply - R3 Button - DUR/PPS Reply and Prior Authorization

The prescription that is referenced appears at the top of the screen with the insurance plan information (Figure 4-25). The *Segment 24 - DUR/PPS Reply* box contains the response to the DUR/PPS Claim. The *DUR/PPS Response Code Counter* box will accept up to nine occurrences. The boxes will be completed by the responder, with reference to up to three different group plans.

The **Reason For Service Code** box will be found in the *Pharmacy Billing Manual for Allowed Values,* and the **Clinical Significance Code** box will indicate the level of significance: 1 for Major, 2 for Moderate, 3 for Minor, and 9 for Undetermined. The box for **Other Pharmacy Indicator** will contain 0 for Not Specified, or 1 for your pharmacy, or 2 for other pharmacy in same chain, or 3 for other pharmacy. The **Previous Date Of Fill** box will contain the date of fill and must be in the CCYYMMDD format. The **Previous Qty Filled** box will contain the amount dispensed.

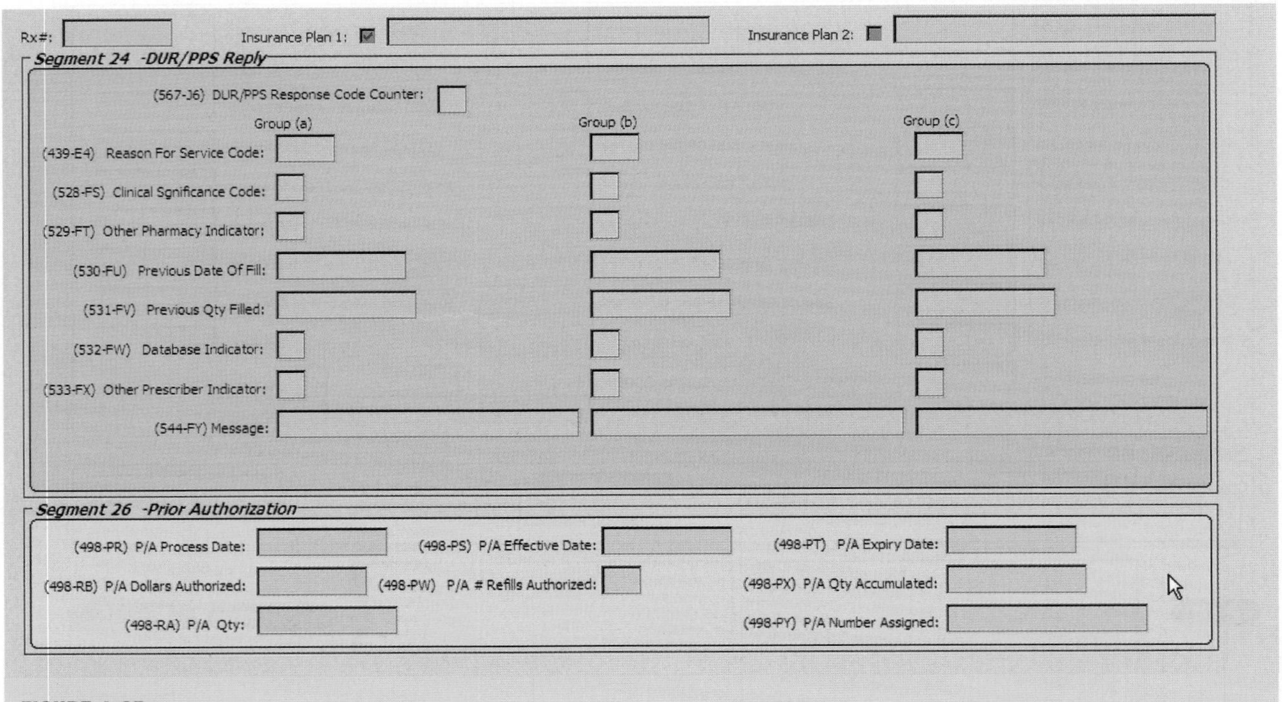

FIGURE 4-25.

The **Database Indicator** box will indicate which database was used for processing the information, such as 1- First DataBank or 4- Processor developed.

The **Other Prescriber Indicator** box indicates by code 1 if it is the same prescriber or 2 for other prescriber. The last line contains three boxes for a **Message** to be written in free-form text if additional clarification is needed.

Segment 26 - Prior Authorization box contains information needed to process dates, dollars authorized, refill information, and prior authorization number. This box is included for future versions of the NCPDP program.

 Note: First DataBank is an information services company that drives patient safety and healthcare quality by providing drug databases within information systems. This company works with customers, pharmacies, to integrate their drug databases to improve user workflow, enhance clinical decision-making at the point-of-need to help reduce the incidence of medication errors and adverse clinical drug events.

EXERCISE I

1. Click on the **Insurance** button in **Main-1** and look at the list of insurance plans in the **Search List** at the bottom of the screen.

2. Perform the following:

   a. Look for the following BIN #'s for Plan Numbers 12, 44, 61, 63, 64, 76, 89, 92, 93, and 172.

   b. List the plan name and BIN #'s.

3. What does NCPDP mean, and what is the mission of NCPDP (*www.ncpdp.org*)?

4. How does a pharmacy establish a working relationship with an insurance company?

EXERCISE II

1. What does AWP mean?

2. What does AAC stand for?

3. What are dispensing units?

4. How are dates entered into the transactions?

5. What are three types of prior authorizations?

EXERCISE III

1. What does DAW mean?

2. What is the meaning of Days Supply?

3. Why do mistakes occur in days supply?

CRITICAL THINKING

1. Why is the BIN entered?

2. Why do you have to verify insurance information with patients, and when would be the best time in the process to verify this information?

3. What are DAW codes, and what do they mean?

4. Why is the correct days supply calculation necessary?

5. What does the abbreviation COB stand for?

6. What does Usual and Customary Charge mean in relation to pricing?

7. In the compound segment of Segment L-10, why does the dosage form code have to match the route of administration code?

8. Drug Utilization Review is used as a way of controlling costs, but it also can be used to provide other valuable information about the patient's medications or services. What is some of this extra information?

9. What is the provider qualifier, and why is it important?

10. In Segment 21 - Status Reply, what information is provided? Why?

CHAPTER 5

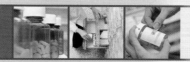

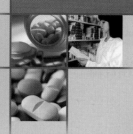

Pricing Table

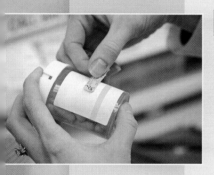

LEARNING OBJECTIVES

1. Explain the purpose of pricing tables.
2. Discuss why changes to pricing tables must be done cautiously.
3. Describe the different types of pricing used in pricing formulas.
4. Explain the function of a pharmacy benefit manager.
5. Explain the wholesaler's position in supplying drugs and supplies.
6. Discuss Average Sales Price and its origin.

Proper pricing is essential for a pharmacy to be profitable. Many factors must be considered when setting up a pricing formula. Pricing is dependent on the actual amount paid for a product, total expense of conducting business, and agreed-upon contractual discounts with customers and insurance providers. Without accurate pricing formulas, a pharmacy may not have control of its costs, profits, and overall business. This chapter takes a quick look at some of the many elements that may go into a pricing formula.

Many factors are involved in pricing a drug or a service, especially considering the type of pharmacy and the type of insurance involved. The pharmacy technician can play a significant role in managing the pricing tables within the pharmacy computer system. Because pricing formulas may originate at the local level for the small independent pharmacy, within a large corporate pharmacy network, or at the institution level, the pharmacist, the pharmacy technician has many different responsibilities in maintaining proper pricing tables.

Pricing tables establish the pricing for the medication or services based on several factors and information that must be entered into the computer system so the proper charges can be processed when a prescription or service is charged to a patient. The **$PriceTbl** button is found

Add PR
Edit
SAVE

Search _____

Price Edit/Create

Price Table Description
AWP - 4% PLUS 3.00

Table Number
60

ROWID
28

Delete

Enter Formula and, if
desired, minimum price
formula.
Use AWP/AAC/MAC/QTY
as variables in formula.

Round Up To   Discount Allowed

Pricing Forumula
AWP * 0.96 + 3.00

Minimum Price Formula (Optional)
.50

Test

Get Current Drug
Record Prices
From Drug Tab
Get Now

TEST VALUES

AWP / Pkg	AAC / Pkg	MAC / Pkg	Units / Package	Sample RX Quan	Price for Sample RX	Amt of Markup
				10.000		

○ Price Table #   ◉ Description

Price Table #	Description	Discount	Round Fact	Price Formula	Minimum Formula
60	AWP - 4% PLUS 3.00~60			AWP * 0.96 + 3.00	5.0
49	CMP10 (AAC * 10 + 2.00)~49	N		AAC * 10 + 2.00	20.0
41	CMP2 (AAC * 2 + 2.00)~41	N		AAC * 2 + 2.00	20.0
42	CMP3 (AAC * 3 + 2.00)~42	N		AAC * 3 + 2.00	20.0
43	CMP4 (AAC * 4 + 2.00)~43	N		AAC * 4 +2.00	20.0

Up

Dn

SELECT RowID, * FROM PriceTbls WHERE [PrcDesc] >= 'AWP - 4% PLUS 3.00~60' ORDER BY [PrcDesc] LIMIT 1

© Apothesoft, LLC.

FIGURE 5-1.

under **Main-1** on the left side of the screen (Figure 5-1). The information entered into this screen is crucial not only from the time the price table is created, but also in maintaining the table with correct information.

At the top of the screen is a **Search** box, which allows for searching for a price table either by description or by the number of the price table. To set which search method will be used, the **Price Table #** or **Description** must be selected above the Search List. Among the other buttons at the top of the screen is the **Add PR** button, which, when selected, will clear the screen and allow for new information to be entered to create a new price table. The **Edit** button allows for the selected price table to be edited for errors or changes in formula. Because making changes to any information in the computer system will affect the prescriptions in the computer system, a **WARNING** box appears as a reminder that *all* changes must be approved by the pharmacist (Figure 5-2).

The **Price Edit/Create** box contains the information about how a price is being created for a medication or service (Figure 5-3). The **Price Table Description** box is intended for the description that will appear in the description column in the Search box at the bottom of the screen. The description can be a short name to represent the type of pricing. For example, pricing a compound with four ingredients could be CMP4. Then the short name would be

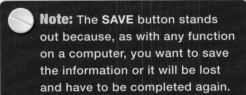

Note: The **SAVE** button stands out because, as with any function on a computer, you want to save the information or it will be lost and have to be completed again.

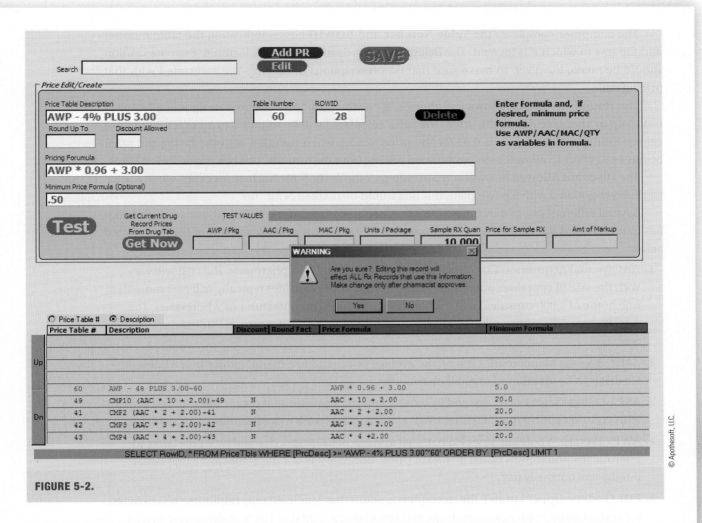

FIGURE 5-2.

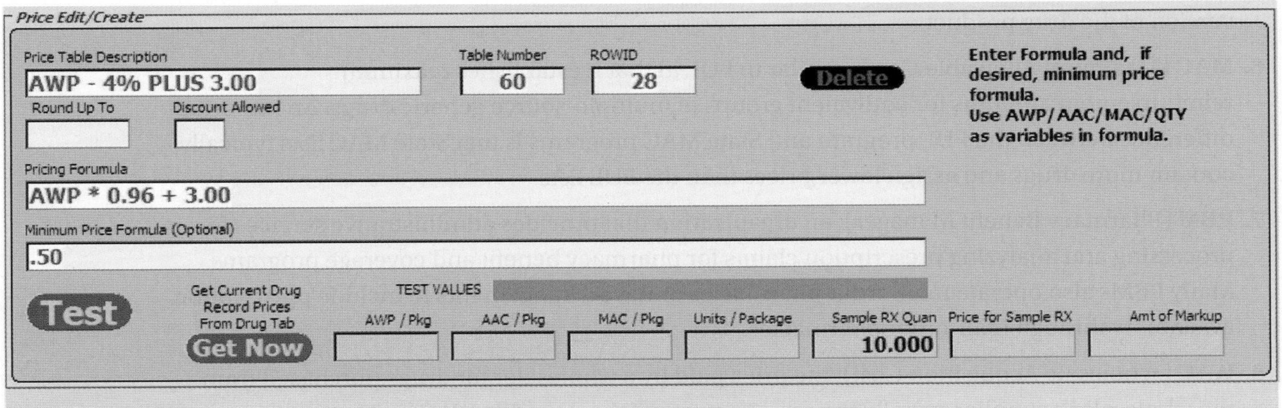

FIGURE 5-3.

followed by the formula used for pricing. For example, CMP4 (AAC × 4 + 2.00) represents the actual acquisition cost times 4 plus $2.00.

The price description also might have a description, such as GEN4 (AAC + 99% + 8.00). This description indicates that the name GEN4 has a price based on actual acquisition cost plus 99% of the AAC plus an $8.00 dispensing fee.

The computer completes the **Table Number** and **ROWID** boxes, indicating the table number and the row in which it is located. The **Delete** button is used to remove a formula. Extreme caution should be taken, however, to make sure that no prescriptions or services are associated with that pricing table.

The **Round Up To** box allows the pharmacist or the corporate office to designate a factor to round up to after calculating the price. The price calculated will be rounded to an exact number of cents. (Example: If the factor is 0.95 for the price $25.33, when rounded with the factor, the price becomes $25.95.) To allow for straightforward pricing from the formula, this box would be left blank.

The **Discount Allowed** box will contain either a Y for Yes or N for No. In most cases, when a price has been negotiated with a payer plan, this box would be marked N for "no".

Several different prices may be used to price medication and services. The pharmacy technician has to understand the various abbreviations used in the pricing formulas. A few of these are listed below:

1. **AAC** (Actual Acquisition Cost): the net cost of a drug paid by a pharmacy. The cost will vary with the size of container purchased (e.g., 5 bottles of 100 capsules typically will cost more than one bottle of 1,000 capsules) and the source of purchase (manufacturer or wholesaler). The AAC includes discounts, rebates, charge-backs, and other adjustments, excluding dispensing fees.

2. **AMP** (Average Manufacturer Price): the average price paid to a manufacturer by a wholesaler for drugs to be distributed to retail pharmacies.

3. **ASP** (Average Sales Price): created by federal and state government prosecutors for settlements with pharmaceutical manufacturers TAP and Bayer to ensure more accurate price reporting.

4. **AWP** (Average Wholesale Price): a national average of list prices charged by wholesalers to pharmacies; sometimes called a "sticker price" because it is not the actual price that larger purchasers normally pay.

5. **FUL** (Federal Upper Limits): the maximum amount that Medicaid may reimburse pharmacies for certain multi-source generic drugs and brand drugs; equal to 150 % of the lowest-priced version of the drug product.

6. **MAC** (Maximum Allowable Cost): similar to FUL in that it establishes maximum reimbursement amounts for equivalent groups of multiple-source generic drugs. An important difference between the FUL program and State MAC programs is that State MAC lists typically contain more drugs and assign lower prices than the FUL lists.

7. **PBM** (Pharmacy Benefit Manager): an organization that provides administrative services for processing and analyzing prescription claims for pharmacy benefit and coverage programs. Many PBMs also operate mail-order pharmacies or have arrangements to include prescription availability through mail-order pharmacies.

8. **WAC** (Wholesale Acquisition Cost): the price paid by a wholesaler for drugs purchased from the wholesaler's supplier, usually the manufacturer of the drug; the WAC amount may not reflect all available discounts.

9. **Wholesaler**: a company that serves as a bridge between the drug manufacturer and a pharmacy or chain of pharmacies; wholesalers do not relabel or repackage the drug.

The **Pricing Formula** box contains the formula used to calculate the price of the drug being dispensed. The Average Wholesale Price (AWP) or Actual Acquisition Cost (AAC) typically is used for calculating the price. Then the price is multiplied by the mark-up percentage factor, such as 60%, which would be entered as a 1.60 factor, or 230%, which would be a 2.30 factor, followed by the addition of the allowable dispensing fee. The dispensing fee is the charge for the professional services provided by the pharmacist when dispensing a prescription. The dispensing fee would include overhead/operating expenses and profit. The dispensing fee does not include cost for the drugs being dispensed. There will always be a variety of different pricing formulas, largely because of the large number of insurance plans, and also negotiated prices with nursing facilities to which the pharmacy may be providing services.

The **Minimum Price Formula (Optional)** box is just that—optional. If the pharmacy decides that a minimum pricing formula is to be used, it would be entered in this box. For instance, if the pricing formula percentage is 0.60 and the minimum percentage is 40%, then 0.40 would be entered as an optional pricing.

The last section, at the bottom of the screen, allows for testing the pricing formula. The **Test** button will indicate to the computer that a test pricing action will be occurring. The **Get Now** button is a shortcut for acquiring the pricing table for the current drug being tested. The **TEST VALUES** box is used for entering a test formula for test price. The following amounts are pulled from the drug screen showing the information for **AWP/Pkg**, **AAC/Pkg**, **MAC/Pkg**, and **Units/Package**. **Sample Rx Quan** can be entered for calculating a price. The sample quantity typically is the usual amount dispensed for a prescription. The **Price for Sample RX** will be calculated and entered in the box. The **Amt of Markup** box will contain how much was made on the drug.

The bottom half of the screen (Figure 5-4) is the **Search List** for the price table. The top of the list box has the designator button to indicate how you want to search for a specific pricing formula, either by **Price Table #** or **Description**, depending on which is checked. You can search for the desired price formula either by using the **Up** and **Dn** (down) buttons or by using the scroll wheel on the mouse.

 Note: When using the Demo version of the program, the **Test** function will not work.

Some pharmacy technicians have an opportunity to attain a job as a Pharmacy Purchasing Agent/Buyer. If so, you would be responsible for procuring supplies, materials, and pharmaceuticals for the pharmacy. In addition, you would maintain computer interface with vendors to ensure procurement of merchandise, reliable delivery, and optimum pricing. You would make sure that the pharmacy has the product and materials on the shelf to supply the patient's needs. You also would be responsible for maintaining inventory records.

As pharmacy technicians begin to play more vital roles within the pharmacy, they have more opportunities and responsibilities to participate in professional organizations such as the National Pharmacy Purchasing Association (*www.pharmacypurchsing.com*) or the National Pharmacy Technician Association (*www.pharmacytechnician.org*).

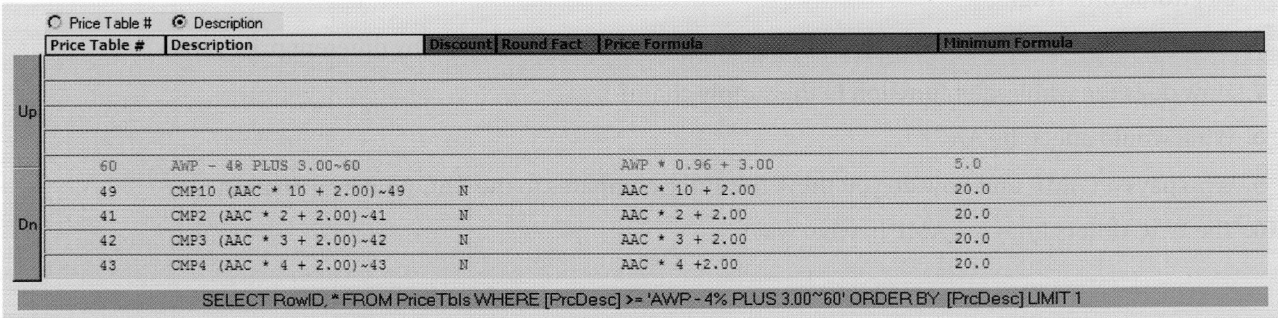

Price Table #	Description	Discount	Round Fact	Price Formula	Minimum Formula
60	AWP - 4% PLUS 3.00~60			AWP * 0.96 + 3.00	5.0
49	CMP10 (AAC * 10 + 2.00)~49	N		AAC * 10 + 2.00	20.0
41	CMP2 (AAC * 2 + 2.00)~41	N		AAC * 2 + 2.00	20.0
42	CMP3 (AAC * 3 + 2.00)~42	N		AAC * 3 + 2.00	20.0
43	CMP4 (AAC * 4 + 2.00)~43	N		AAC * 4 +2.00	20.0

(○ Price Table #   ◉ Description)

SELECT RowID, * FROM PriceTbls WHERE [PrcDesc] >= 'AWP - 4% PLUS 3.00~60' ORDER BY [PrcDesc] LIMIT 1

FIGURE 5-4.

© Apothesoft, LLC.

EXERCISE I

1. Look up the website *www.rxinsider.com* to find wholesalers, and list at least five. After listing the wholesalers, write a brief description of each.

2. Look up the website *www.pharmacychoice.com* and find the wholesalers list. List the wholesalers that differ from the wholesalers you listed above.

3. What is one difference between MAC pricing and FUL pricing?

4. What is included in the Price Table Description?

5. What are the components of the Pricing Formula?

EXERCISE II

1. Scroll through the Price Table **Search List** and look at the various descriptions. What do the four-letter descriptions preceding the pricing formulas represent?

2. Looking at the descriptions, what is the difference between the price tables using AWP and those using AAC as the drug cost to calculate the pricing formula?

3. The price table has a pricing description starting with "CMP". What does the number at the end of "CMP" represent in the description and the formula?

4. How would you use the Round Up To function in the Pricing Table?

5. How would you search for a specific pricing formula?

CRITICAL THINKING

1. What are some of the many responsibilities of a pharmacy purchaser?

2. Why do you think it is important to belong to a professional organization?

3. Other than for recertification, why should you do more than just read CE (Continuing Education) material and take the tests?

4. If working as a pharmacy purchaser, how would you make sure that the pricing information is correct?

5. Many vendors interface directly with the pharmacy for electronic ordering. What are the advantages of electronic ordering?

6. Looking at the Price Table **Search List**, why do you think there are so many different price tables?

7. How does the wholesaler function in the supply chain?

8. What would affect the AAC?

9. Who pays an AMP, and how do you think this price compares to the AAC paid by a pharmacy?

10. The WAC differs from the AMP in what way?

CHAPTER **6**

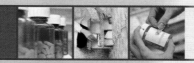

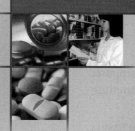

Inputting Compounds

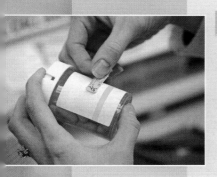

LEARNING OBJECTIVES

1. Indicate where to locate NDC numbers if they are not available.

2. Discuss the type of information needed for the package and price information.

3. Explain the type of components that make up the intravenous compound.

4. Explain the NDC for the compound and why is it different from a regular manufacturer's NDC number.

5. Explain how the sig codes for intravenous compounds are different from a sig code for an oral medication.

Maintaining intravenous compounds in the pharmacy inventory and compounding must be handled properly to ensure proper billing, correct medications, and intravenous fluids as well as patient safety. Although intravenous compounding does not require as many ingredients to be combined, they do require different sig codes and directions. This chapter covers the process of entering intravenous compounds into the pharmacy computer system compound screen and how these differ from extemporaneous compounds.

At times, the pharmacy will receive a prescription order for a medication or a specific form of a medication that is not available commercially. These orders require the pharmacy to compound the medication or change the medication to a different form for administration. The pharmacy then does what is known as *compounding*. The two types of compounding are sterile and non-sterile. Sterile compounding requires clean room facilities and aseptic manipulations of products.

Pharmacy technicians sometimes are called upon to make compounds. This will depend on the pharmacy's policy and the pharmacy technician's skill and knowledge. Some pharmacy technicians learn compounding while attending a pharmacy technician formal training class. Other technicians have learned on the job or completed a compounding program that offers certification in compounding. Professional organizations such as the NPTA (National Pharmacy Technician Association) or companies that specialize in supplying compounding materials and equipment such as the PCCA (Professional Compounding Center of America) offer these training programs for technicians.

Compounding requires the use of a detailed formula that contains directions on how to prepare, store, and label the final compound. The pharmacy maintains records of the compound to include the ingredients' NDC numbers and lot numbers with expiration dates.

For pricing the compound and for processing the charge for the compound through an insurance payer, the compound ingredients must be in the pharmacy computer system. The pharmacist or the pharmacy technician will have to enter those ingredients in the **Compound Formula** screen.

ENTERING A COMPOUND FORMULA

To access the **Compounding Formula** box, you must be in the **Main-1** screen. Then select the **Dg-Scrn** button on the left side of the screen (Figure 6-1).

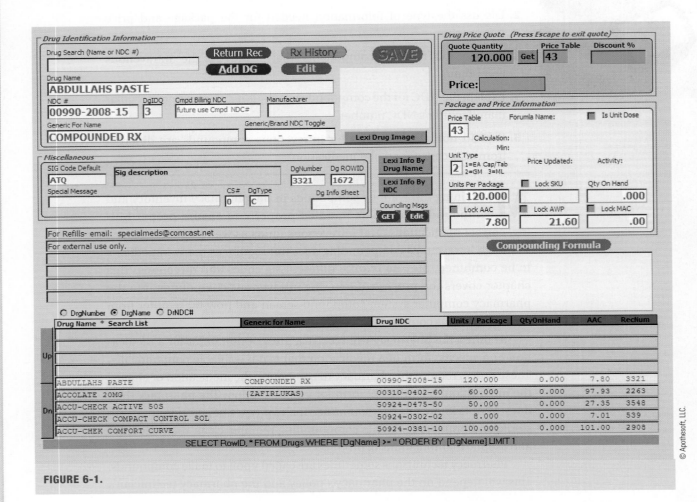

FIGURE 6-1.

© Apothesoft, LLC.

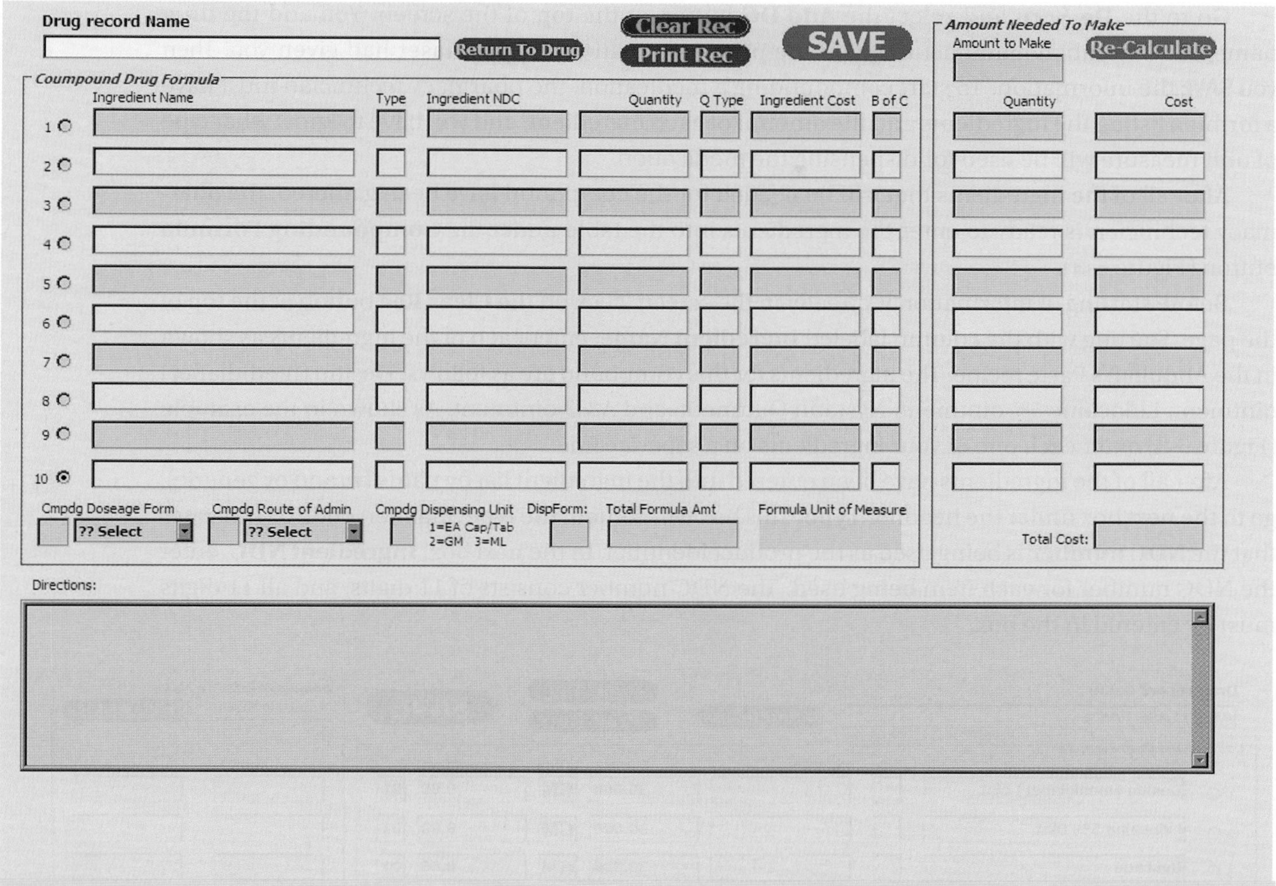

FIGURE 6-2.

When the **Dg-Scrn** box opens, the **Compounding Formula** button above a blank box is located on the right side of the drug box under the ***Package and Price Information*** box. Click on the **Compounding Formula** button (Figure 6-2) to open the ***Compound Drug Formula*** screen.

This screen contains the ingredients for the compound listed in the **Drug record Name** box. The ingredients listed for that compound must be listed in the **Drug Name Search List** before they can be added to the **Ingredient Name** list. Check the **Drug Name Search List** for all the ingredients before entering the name of the drug to be compounded. If all of the ingredients do not appear in the drug list, you will have to enter the ingredients into **Dg-Scrn** screen.

Assume that you have received an order for Abdullah's Paste, which does not appear in the **Drug Name Search List**, so it must be entered into the computer system. Scroll through the **Drug Name Search List** and check for each ingredient. You find everything in the compound formula recipe except Nystatin Ointment 10,0000 units/gram. You check the shelf for the Nystatin, but it is not in stock. Then you check with the pharmacy purchaser and find that the 30-gram tubes of Nystatin Ointment 10,0000 units/gram have just come in with the drug delivery. The Nystatin is a new item for the pharmacy and must be entered into the inventory in the computer.

The pharmacy purchaser is busy, so you have to compound the Abdullah's Paste. You volunteer to enter the Nystatin Ointment, and the pharmacy purchaser allows you to help with entering the Nystatin Ointment.

Go to the **Dg-Scrn** and select the **Add DG** button at the top of the screen. You add the drug name, NDC number, manufacturer, and the price information the purchaser had given you. Then you **SAVE** the information. To start compounding a medication, the pharmacy technician must have a formula listing the ingredients and the amount of each ingredient, and will have to know what type of unit measure will be used for dispensing the medication.

After all of the ingredients that will be needed for the compound have been gathered, the pharmacy technician is ready to enter the ingredients into the table under the **Compounding Formula** button (Figure 6-3).

Before starting, if information is already in the screen, click on the **Clear Rec** button at the top of the page. Starting with the column labeled **Ingredient Name**, enter each of the ingredients as shown in the Abdullah's Paste recipe. The ingredients for this compound are as follows: Desitin (medidiaper) ointment, Lidocaine 5% ointment, Nystatin Ointment, and A&D ointment. As shown in the example (Figure 6-3) enter each one of your ingredients on a separate line.

After all of the ingredients have been entered into the ingredient list by name (brand or generic), go to the next box under the heading **Type.** This box will contain the type qualifier; code 03 indicates that the **NDC number** is being used as the product identifier. In the next box, **Ingredient NDC**, enter the NDC number for each item being used. The NDC number consists of 11 digits, and all 11 digits must be entered in the box.

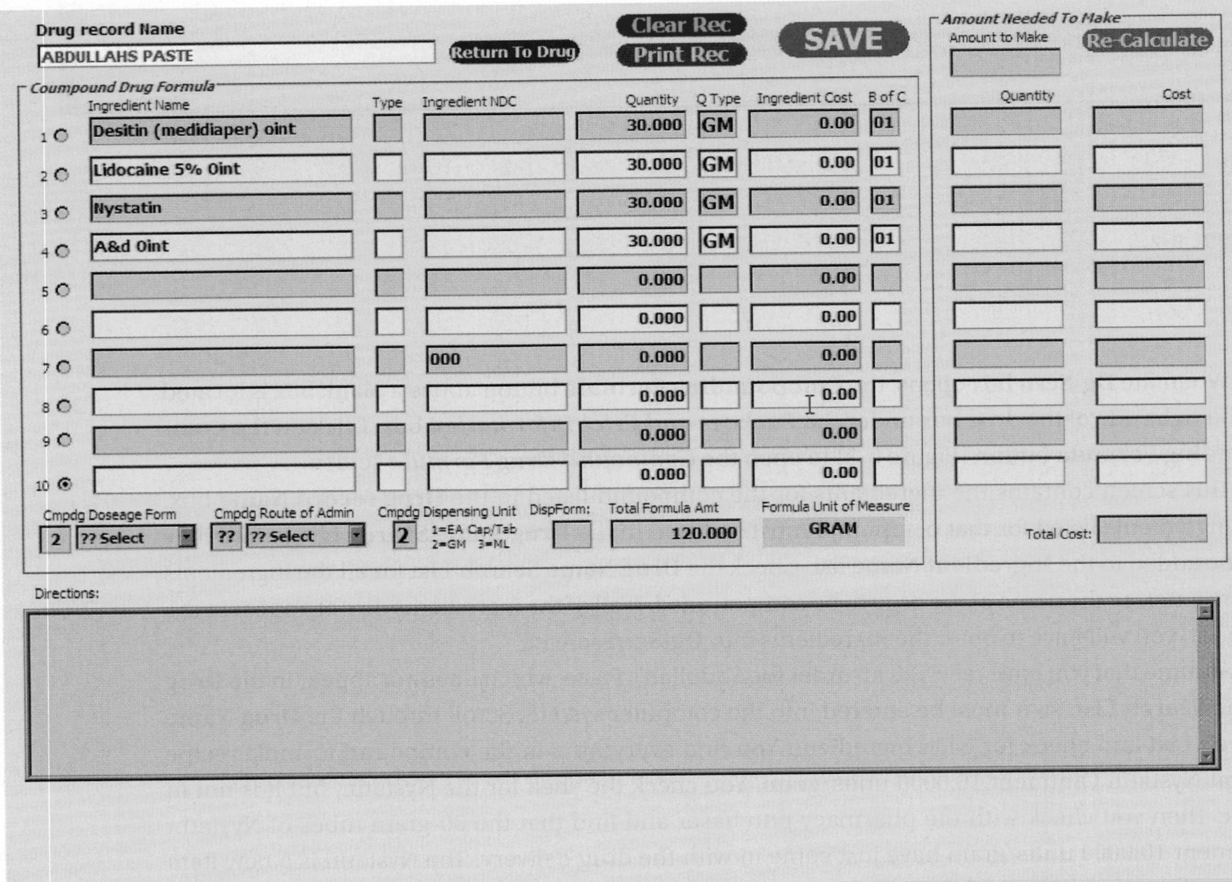

FIGURE 6-3.

© Apothesoft, LLC.

The next box is for indicating the **Quantity**, which indicates how much of the ingredient is being used in this compound. In the **Q Type** box, enter the type of measurement being used to determine the quantity amount. Be sure to use the appropriate quantity type: MG=Milligrams, GM=Grams, ML=Milliliters, MC=Micrograms, OZ=Ounces, LB=Pounds, and EA=Each. In this formula, you are using GM for all of the quantity types.

In the next box, **Ingredient Cost**, you will have to make sure that the correct amount is charged for the compound. A pharmacy technician who is given the responsibility of making sure that all compounds are being priced correctly will have to check this regularly. This is also true for any new compounds added into the computer system. Remember that the cost of ingredients can change quickly because of substitute items and price increases from the supplier, as well as the cost of the containers for dispensing.

 Note: Be sure to check with the pharmacist before making any changes to the cost.

The next box, the **B of C** (Basis of Cost Determination), normally will default to 01 for AWP (Average Wholesale Price).

Across the bottom of the *Compound Drug Formula* box are two boxes that have drop-down boxes next to them for **Cmpdg Dosage Form** and **Cmpdg Route of Admin** to indicate the form of the compounded drug and how it will be administered. The next box, **Cmpdg Dispensing Unit**, indicates the compounded units being dispensed. The **DispForm** box code will use the same codes as the previous box to indicate the form of the compound. The **Total Formula Amt** box represents the sum of the amounts shown in the above **Quantity** boxes. The **Formula Unit of Measure** box indicates the formula dispensing form.

At the bottom of the screen is a **Directions** box (Figure 6-4) for indicating, in free-form text, the directions of use and any additional information which the pharmacy may need to include on the label.

To the far right of the ingredients is an Amount Needed To Make box that allows for an easy way of recalculating the cost, if the prescription requires making a larger or smaller amount of the compounded medication. In the **Amount to Make** box, enter the amount that has been compounded, click the **Re-Calculate** button, and the program will re-calculate the amounts needed and the new cost.

One of the useful buttons at the top of the screen is the **Print Rec** button. Once you have entered all of the ingredients and the corresponding information, you may print out a record or just view it on the screen before printing to make sure you have entered everything properly. After you have printed out the record, you can save the record in a binder for future reference. The printed record will show only the ingredients used and the amount of each ingredient.

Directions:

Use as directed by physician.

© Apothesoft, LLC.

FIGURE 6-4.

EXERCISE I

Using the compound below or one you have made in class or at work, enter the ingredients for the compound into the compounding screen. Be sure to check the drug **Search List** first. If the drug is not in the list, add it to the drug screen.

Notice that Magic Mouthwash has more than one name. Also, it has several recipes because the prescriber will prescribe what it wants to go into the mouthwash.

Supply List Info:

Diphenhydramine Elixir 12.5 mg/5 mL 473 mL bottle   00603-0823-54
    Qualitest $13.01

Maalox   150ml bottle   00067-0330-62   Novartis $ 2.73

Viscous Lidocaine 2%   100 mL bottle   00054-35000-49
    Roxane Laboratories $13.99

> **Magic Mouthwash Recipe 2 (also called "Xyloxadryl" or "BMX")**
>
> *Rx:*
> - *1 Part viscous lidocaine 2%*
> - *1 Part Maalox (do not substitute Kaopectate)*
> - *1 Part diphenhydramine 12.5 mg per 5 mL elixir*
>
> *Quantity: 120 mL*
> *Sig: Swish, gargle, and spit one to two teaspoonfuls every six hours as needed. May be swallowed if esophageal involvement.*

EXERCISE II

Looking at the above prescription for the Magic Mouthwash, how much of each of the ingredients will be entered in the **Quantity** column?

EXERCISE III

Looking at the above prescription, enter the cost of each ingredient. Are you entering the cost of the entire container or the amount being used? How do you calculate the cost of the amount being used?

EXERCISE IV

Select what **Cmpdg Dosage Form** is being compounded and the **Cmpdg Route of Admin**.

CRITICAL THINKING

1. When entering compounds, what first steps should you take, especially if a recipe is not entered already into the compounding formula screen?

2. Where can you find an NDC number for a specific drug? List all of the different sources that provide this information.

3. When selecting the product off the shelf to use in the compound, what should you take into consideration in relation to the size of the product?

4. What type of information would you enter in the **Directions** box?

5. Where can a pharmacy technician learn how to compound?

6. How would you use the **Re-Calculate** button?

7. When entering ingredients for a compound, many steps must be followed to ensure accuracy of the compound. List these steps for entering a compound into the computer.

8. What information is kept in a written record for each compounded drug?

9. Why should you check the ingredients and prices in the compounds occasionally?

10. Why is compounding done, and how many different forms of compounded medications are you familiar with?

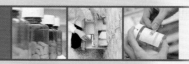

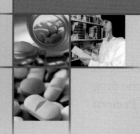

CHAPTER 7

Entering Intravenous Medication Compounds

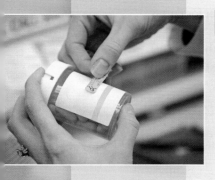

LEARNING OBJECTIVES

1. Indicate where to locate NDC numbers if they are not available.

2. Discuss the type of information needed for the package and price information.

3. Explain the type of components that make up the intravenous compound.

4. Explain the NDC for the compound and why is it different from the ingredient NDC.

5. Explain how the sig codes for intravenous compounds are different from sig codes for other medications.

Maintaining intravenous compounds in the pharmacy inventory and compounding must be handled properly to ensure proper billing, correct medications, and intravenous fluids as well as patient safety. Although intravenous compounding does not require as many ingredients to be combined, they do require different sig codes and directions. This chapter covers the process of entering intravenous compounds into the pharmacy computer system compound screen and how these differ from extemporaneous compounds.

Various programs are available for entering intravenous compound orders. The discussion in Chapter 6 addressed how to enter compounds. All intravenous medication orders are compounds because the prescribed medication is being combined with a prescribed intravenous fluid.

Injectable medications usually are entered into the computer system by the pharmacy purchaser/buyer. In some practice settings, however, the pharmacy technician is responsible for compounding these medications into intravenous fluids, which requires close attention.

ENTERING INJECTABLE MEDICATIONS

After receiving a prescription order for an intravenous medication, search the drug list by clicking on the **Dg-Scrn** button to check for the ordered medication (Figure 7-1). If the medication is in the drug list, you can proceed with entering the order. Return to the patient screen by clicking on the **Pt-Scrn** button (Figure 7-2).

If the medication and intravenous fluid do not appear on the drug list, enter the medication and the intravenous fluid into the drug list before proceeding to the **Compounding Formula** box on the drug screen. In most cases, a pharmacist or a pharmacy technician is responsible for entering all of the medications and compounds in the system. Any technician working in the pharmacy, however, may be called upon to handle this responsibility. Therefore, you should become familiar with the process of entering medications into the drug list. Whether the order is a single order or an admission sheet with multiple orders, it is always handled the same way. For example: You have received the following order for Fortaz 1 gram in 50 mL NS infuse over 30 minutes q12hrs.

Click on the **Dg-Scrn** button. The drug screen will open (Figure 7-3). You can search the drug list quickly by typing the first few letters of the drug, such as "FOR", and the drug **Search List** will go to the drugs starting with the letter "F." Fortaz does not appear in the drug list.

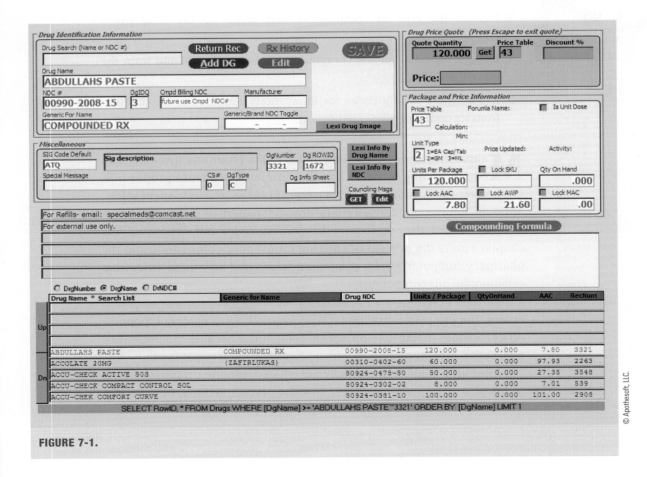

FIGURE 7-1.

© Apothesoft, LLC.

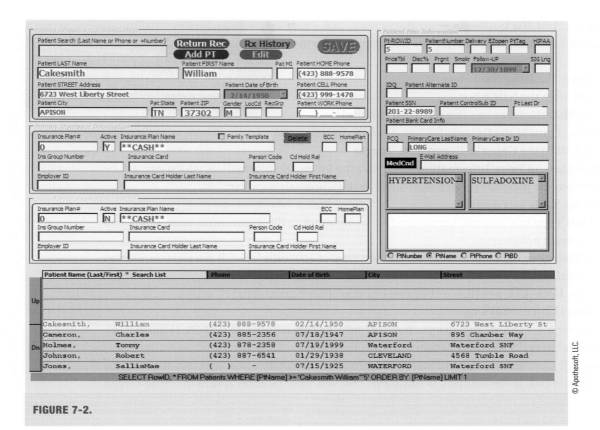

FIGURE 7-2.

FIGURE 7-3.

© Apothesoft, LLC.

Click on the **Add DG** button to clear the screen, and enter the following information in the **Drug Identification Information** box:

Fortaz 1Gm in the **Drug Name** box

00173-0378-10 in the **NDC#** box

GSK in the **Manufacturer** box (for GlaxoSmithKline)

(Ceftazidime 1 gm) in the Generic for Name box

00069-0011-01 in the **Generic/Brand NDC Toggle**

In the **Package and Price Information** box, enter the following information, which you will be able to obtain from the pharmacy purchaser/buyer or the wholesale supplier:

1 in the **Price Table** as a default

3 in the **Unit Type** box (use mL because, when compounding the intravenous compound, you will be using milliliters)

100 in the **Units Per Package** box (there will be a total of 100 units [mLs] if the vials are diluted with 10mLs each)

151.10 in the **Lock AAC** box (this is the price of a tray of 10–1 gram vials)

Don't forget to click on the **SAVE** button!

Do the same for each of the drugs that you add to the computer system (Figure 7-4). Again—remember to verify the information with the pharmacist.

Now you will have to look for the sterile solution for the medication delivery that will be used in the compound. If the solution is not there, you will have to enter it into the drug screen (Figure 7-5).

> **Note:** If you need to find an NDC number for a drug, go to *www.hipaaspace.com* and select NDC Lookup from the list of services.

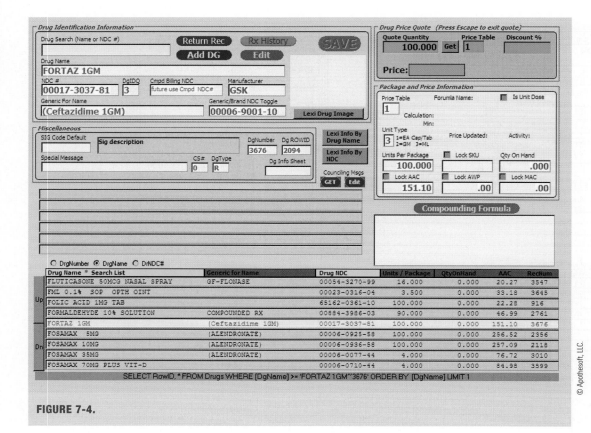

FIGURE 7-4.

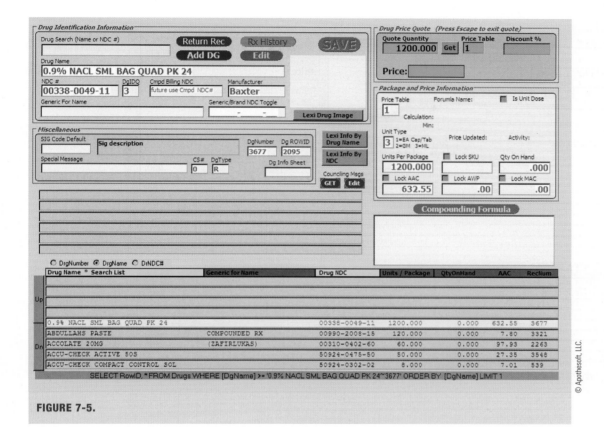

FIGURE 7-5.

© Apothesoft, LLC.

0.9% NaCl 50 mL bag Quad Pk 24 in the **Drug Name** box
00338-0049-11 in the **NDC #** box
Baxter in the **Manufacturer** box

In the **Package and Price Information** box, enter the following information, which you will be able to obtain from the pharmacy purchaser/buyer or the wholesale supplier:

1 in the **Price Table** as a default

3 in the **Unit Type** box (use mL because when compounding the intravenous compound, you will be using milliliters)

1200.000 in the **Units Per Package** box (there will be a total of 50 units [mLs] in each bag in a case of 24)

632.55 in the **Lock ACC** box (this is the price of a case of 24–50 mL bags)

As always, remember to click on the **SAVE** button.

After making sure that the required medications and solutions appear in the drug screen, it is time to enter the I.V. compound. Before entering the ingredients in the compound, though, enter the compound in the **Dg-Scrn** and use the **NDC # 00999-9999-99** for the compound (Figure 7-6).

In the **Dg-Scrn**, click on the **Compounding Formula** button to open the compound screen. This is where you will enter the intravenous compound information. At the compound screen, you will notice that the name for the compound you just entered into the **Dg-Scrn** appears in the **Drug record Name** box and that the **Ingredient Name** column is blank (Figure 7-7).

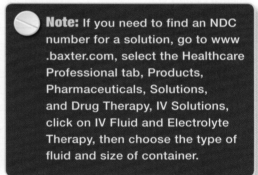

Note: If you need to find an NDC number for a solution, go to www.baxter.com, select the Healthcare Professional tab, Products, Pharmaceuticals, Solutions, and Drug Therapy, IV Solutions, click on IV Fluid and Electrolyte Therapy, then choose the type of fluid and size of container.

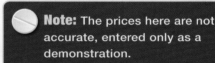

Note: The prices here are not accurate, entered only as a demonstration.

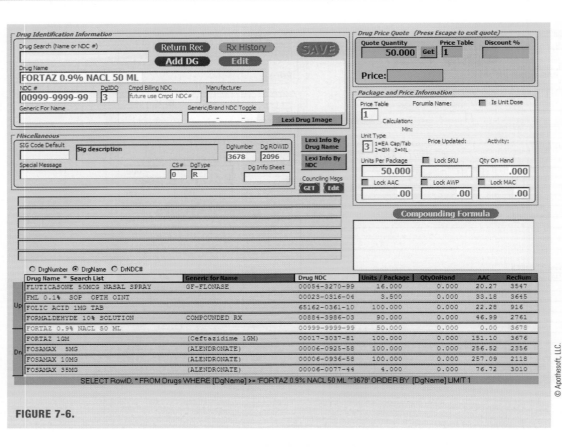

FIGURE 7-6.

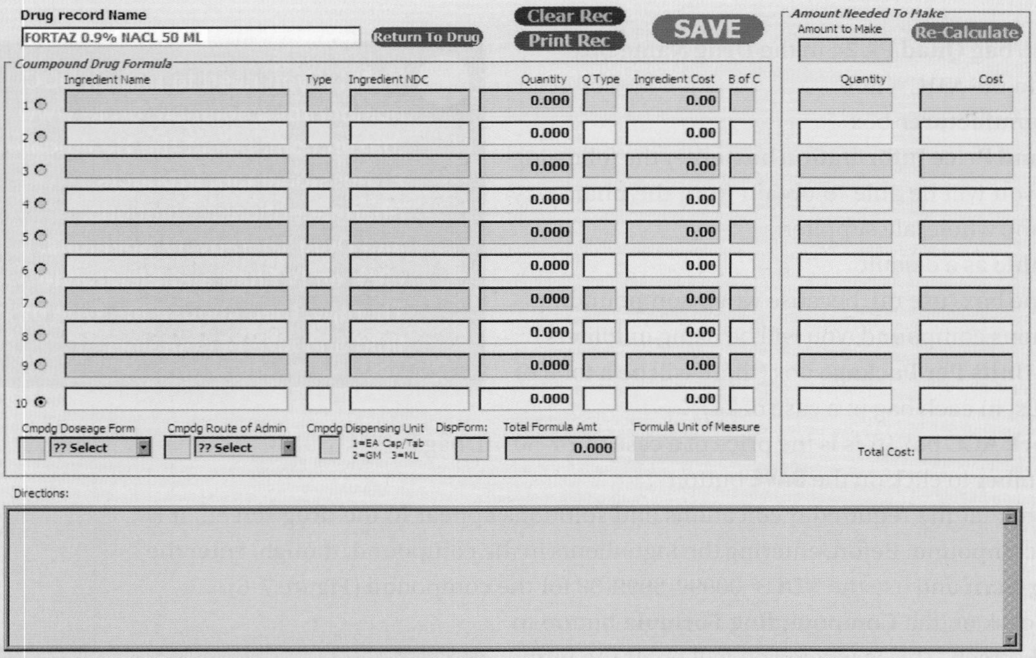

FIGURE 7-7.

© Apothesoft, LLC.

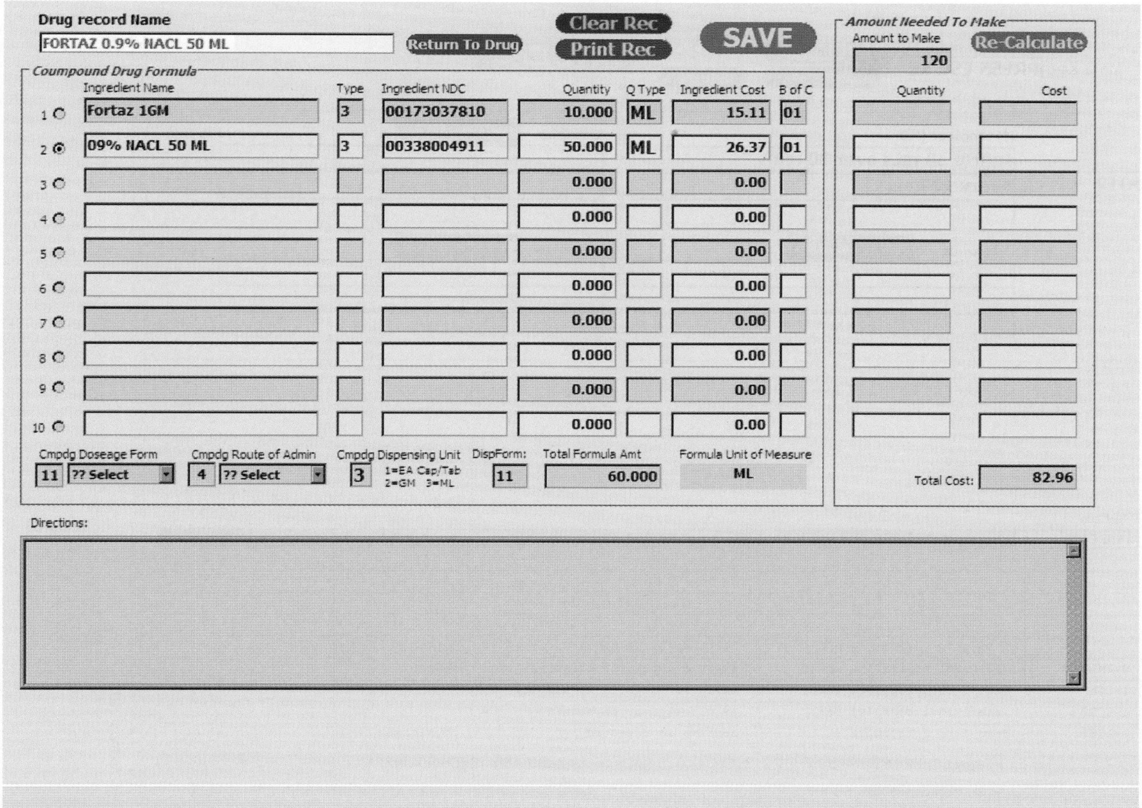

FIGURE 7-8.

Starting with the medication, enter **Fortaz 1 GM** and **0.9% NACL** 50 mL (Figure 7-8). Next, enter the code **03** under **Type** and the NDC number for each in the **Ingredient NDC** column. In the **Quantity** column, enter the amount of each ingredient you are going to use. The 1-gram vial of Fortaz will be reconstituted with 10 mLs of 0.9% sodium chloride for injection, so 10 mLs would be entered for the quantity. The volume of 50 mLs would be entered for the 0.9% sodium chloride bag.

In the **Q Type** column, enter mL for milliliters, and for the **Ingredient Cost**, enter the cost for one vial of Fortaz and one bag of 0.9% sodium chloride. Now remember to select the **Cmpdg Dosage Form**, **Cmpdg Route of Admin**, **Cmpdg Dispensing Unit**, **DispForm**, **Total Formula Amt**, and **Formula Unit of Measure**.

You can calculate the cost of the compound in the **Amount Needed To Make** section. When you enter **120** in the **Amount to Make** box, the cost of two bags of Fortaz will be calculated. Remember to enter the prescription information in the **Directions** box: **Infuse 50 mL over 30 minutes every 12 hours** (Figure 7-8). And, of course, click on the **SAVE** button.

Again, orders for intravenous compounds require different sig directions and codes. These directions should include the volume to infuse over a given amount of time. This should be kept in mind when developing a sig code. The new sig codes are entered by clicking on the **Sig-Scrn** button in the **Main-1** menu (Figure 7-9). When developing a sig code, try to make a code that is easy to remember. For example, **50I30Q12** represents **Infuse** 50 mLs over 30 minutes every 12 hours. The 50 is entered first to make it easy to find in the sig list and is separated from the "over 30 minutes" by the "I" for infuse.

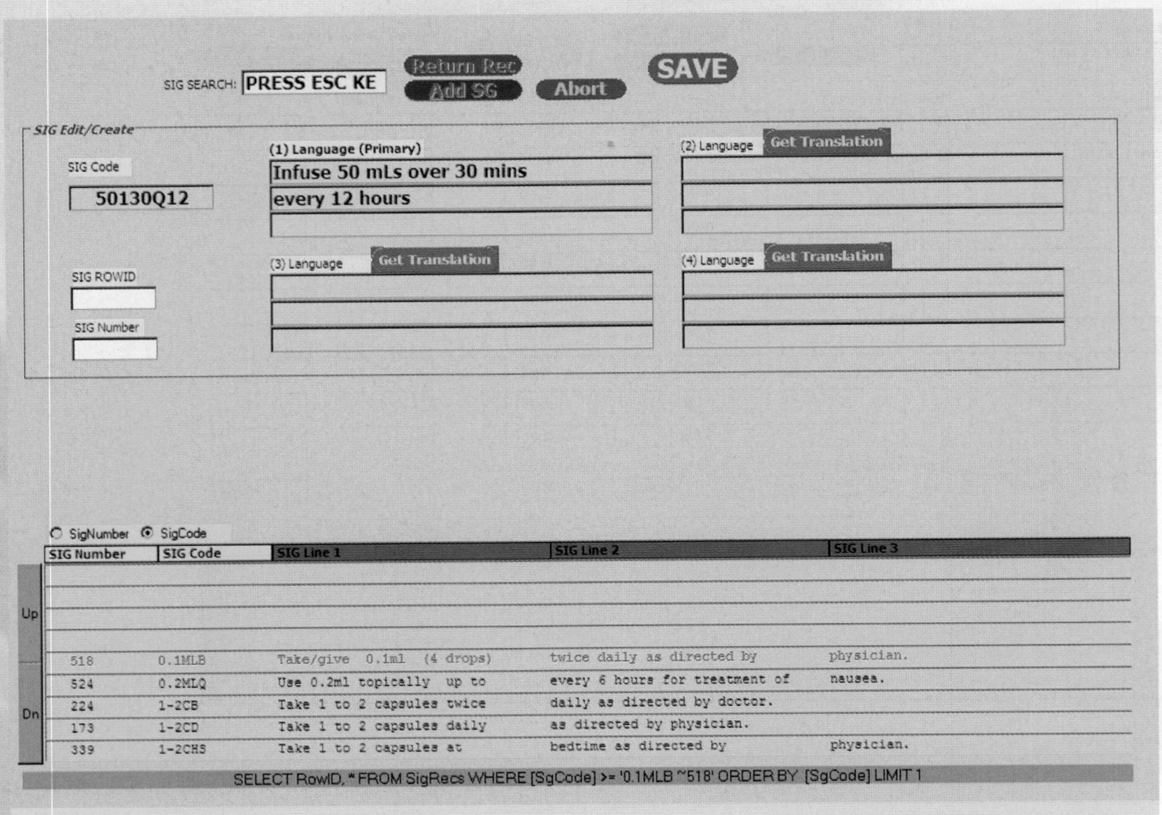

SIG SEARCH: **PRESS ESC KE**   Return Rec   Add SG   Abort   **SAVE**

SIG Edit/Create

SIG Code

50130Q12

SIG ROWID

SIG Number

(1) Language (Primary)

Infuse 50 mLs over 30 mins
every 12 hours

(2) Language   Get Translation

(3) Language   Get Translation

(4) Language   Get Translation

○ SigNumber ◉ SigCode

SIG Number	SIG Code	SIG Line 1	SIG Line 2	SIG Line 3
518	0.1MLB	Take/give 0.1ml (4 drops)	twice daily as directed by	physician.
524	0.2MLQ	Use 0.2ml topically up to	every 6 hours for treatment of	nausea.
224	1-2CB	Take 1 to 2 capsules twice	daily as directed by doctor.	
173	1-2CD	Take 1 to 2 capsules daily	as directed by physician.	
339	1-2CHS	Take 1 to 2 capsules at	bedtime as directed by	physician.

SELECT RowID, * FROM SigRecs WHERE [SgCode] >= '0.1MLB "518' ORDER BY [SgCode] LIMIT 1

© Apothesoft, LLC.

FIGURE 7-9.

After you have entered the compound, have a pharmacist check it. As a pharmacy technician entering intravenous medication orders, you must be able to concentrate and give attention to detail to ensure that all of the proper pieces come together. Keep patient safety and well-being in mind at all times. Although the pharmacist has the primary responsibility for making the final inspection of the compounded intravenous medication, pharmacy technicians are also responsible for the intravenous medication they have compounded.

EXERCISE I

Review Chapters 6 and 7 on Inputting Inventory and Inputting Compounds. List the steps for entering a medication and an intravenous fluid that does not appear in the drug inventory.

EXERCISE II

In some practice settings, such as long-term care pharmacies and home health, supplies must be sent with the intravenous medications. Discuss and list the type of supplies that the nursing staff or the patient would have to set up and administer the intravenous medication. Visit a website such as *www.medicalsuppliesexpert.com* to help you with your list.

EXERCISE III

Enter the following intravenous medication compounds and sig codes:

MEDICATION	INTRAVENOUS FLUID	INFUSE RATE
Ancef (Cefazolin) 1 GM	Sodium Chloride 0.9%	50 mL over 30 minutes
Fortaz (Ceftazidime) 1GM	Sodium Chloride 0.9%	50 mL over 30 minutes
Gentamicin 40 mg	Sodium Chloride 0.9%	50 mL over 30 minutes
Maxipime (Cefepime HCL) 1 GM	Sodium Chloride 0.9%	50 mL over 30 minutes
Nafcillin 1GM	Sodium Chloride 0.9%	50 mL over 30 minutes
Piperacillin 2.5 GM	Sodium Chloride 0.9%	100 mL over 30 minutes
Timentin (Ticarcillin/Clavulonic Acid) 3.1 GM	Sodium Chloride 0.9%	100 mL over 30 minutes
Tobramycin 60 mg	Sodium Chloride 0.9%	100 mL over 45 minutes
Vancomycin 250 mg	Dextrose 5% Sterile Water	100 mL over 30 minutes
Zosyn (Piperacillin/Tazobactam) 3.375 GM	Sodium Chloride 0.9%	100 mL over 30 minutes

MEDICATION INFORMATION

The following information will be used to enter the medications into the system:

Ancef (Cefazolin)–1 gram vials–25 10mL vials per box–NDC# 00007-3130-16 GlaxoSmithKline

$84.00 per box of 25 vials

Store: 24 hours at room temperature–10 days refrigerated - LABEL: Refrigerate

Fortaz (Ceftazidime)–1 gram vials - 10 vials per tray–NDC# 00173-0378-10 GlaxoSmithKline

$151.10 per box of 25 vials

Store: 1 day at room temperature–7 days refrigerated–LABEL: Refrigerate

Gentamicin–40 mg/mL–25 2mL–vials per box–NDC# 00409-1207-03 Hospira

$22.79 per box of 25 vials

Store: 1 day at room temperature–4 days refrigerated–LABEL: Refrigerate

Nafcillin–1 gram vials–10 vials per package–NDC# 00781-3128-92 Sandoz, Inc.

$147.50 per package of 10 vials

Store: 24 hours at room temperature–96 hours refrigerated–LABEL: Refrigerate

Maxipime (Cefepime HCL)–1 gram–10 15mL vials per tray–NDC# 51479-054-30 Bristol-Myers Squibb

$218.30 per tray of 10 vials

Store: 24 hours at room temperature–7 days refrigerated - LABEL: Refrigerate

Piperacillin–3-gram vials–10 vials per box–NDC# 0206-3882-55
Wyeth Pharmaceuticals

$124.00 per box of 10 vials

Store: 1 day at room temperature–7 days refrigerated–LABEL:
Refrigerate

Timentin (Ticarcillin/Clavulonic Acid)–3.1-gram vial–10 vials per
tray–NDC# 00029-6571-40 GlaxoSmithKline

$159.99 per tray of 10 vials

Store: 1 at room temperature–3 days refrigerated–LABEL: Refrigerate

Tobramycin–40mg/mL–25 2mL–vials in tray–NDC# 00409-3578-01–Hospira

$27.97 per tray of 25 vials

Store: 1 day at room temperature–2 days refrigerated–LABEL: Refrigerate

Vancomycin - 1-gram vial–25 vials per package–NDC# 00409-6533-01–Hospira

$67.40 per package of 10 vials

Store: 2 days at room temperature–14 days refrigerated–LABEL: Refrigerate

Zosyn: 3.375 gram vial–10 vials per tray–NDC# 00206-8854-16 Wyeth Pharmaceuticals

$236.15 per tray of 10 vials

Store: 1 day at room temperature–7 days refrigerated–LABEL: Refrigerate

 Note: For additional information on dilutions and usage of intravenous medications, refer to the Globalrph website, *www.globalrph.com*

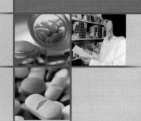

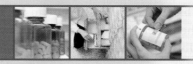

CHAPTER 8

Entering Prescriptions

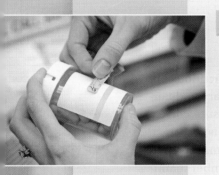

LEARNING OBJECTIVES

1. Demonstrate the ability to enter patient information into a computer system.
2. Illustrate knowledge of what information is required in the computer system.
3. Discuss the importance of attention to detail when entering patients and prescriptions.
4. Practice accuracy as well as speed when entering patient information into the computer system.
5. Discuss the importance of selecting the correct patient's physician when entering prescriptions.

Entering patient information into the pharmacy computer system is the initial task that must be accomplished before the patient's prescriptions, treatments, and pharmacy supply orders can be completed. This requires attention to detail to prevent medication errors as well as to make sure that the patient is charged correctly, the correct doctor is associated with the order, and the pharmacy is compensated properly for services. This chapter provides the opportunity to practice your skills in entering patients, physicians, and prescriptions.

In most practice settings, the one certain activity that the pharmacy technician will be performing is to enter patient information and prescriptions. In this chapter, we offer practice for you to enter patient information and prescriptions into the computer system. In entering the prescriptions, you may have to refer to the patient information in Appendix C. Refer back to previous chapters if you need help in entering these prescriptions.

When entering the patient information, keep in mind that if you pay close attention to detail, you will not make medication errors and also will ensure that the patient will be billed accurately. Be sure to ask the patient about any allergies, as this information can prevent the patient from having an adverse or life-threatening reaction to a prescribed medication. Appendix C includes a sample patient information sheet.

In some cases, you may have to enter a new drug. In most work settings, a pharmacy technician serves as the pharmacy or corporate purchaser/buyer who is responsible for entering new medications. In any case, pharmacy technicians should be aware of what has to be done to enter new drugs or supplies into the computer system. If the drug does not appear in the drug **Search List**, the drug will have to be entered into the drug screen before completing the prescription.

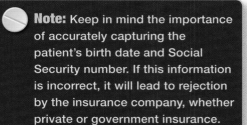

Note: Keep in mind the importance of accurately capturing the patient's birth date and Social Security number. If this information is incorrect, it will lead to rejection by the insurance company, whether private or government insurance.

Again, pay close attention to the correct spelling of the patient's name, the correct medication, and the directions for taking or using the medication. Also, make sure when selecting the prescribed medication to select the correct form and strength.

DRUG ENFORCEMENT ADMINISTRATION NUMBER VERIFICATION PROCESS

The DEA numbers on the prescription for each of the physicians in this chapter are fictitious but do contain the correct alpha and numeric configuration. The DEA number is necessary to determine if the prescriber is allowed to prescribe scheduled medications and also to assure correct insurance billing. At times, an insurance claim is rejected because the DEA number is incorrect. Today's pharmacy software systems are programmed to check the DEA number to make sure it is accurate, but the pharmacy technician still must know how to check the DEA number manually when the computer system is down or if the insurance claim requires a follow-up. Therefore, when re-checking all of the information for the insurance claim, quickly check the DEA number manually.

In addition, the pharmacy manager might subscribe to an organization that provides physician DEA numbers and other license information. You also may check these sites but still check the numbers manually as a double-check.

Assume that you have received a prescription from Dr. Doug Lowell for Percocet 5/325. Dr. Lowell's DEA number is BL2455562. To verify that this is the correct DEA number for Dr. Lowell, check the following manually:

1. Make sure the first letter is either A, B, or M.

2. Make sure the second letter is the first letter in the last name. In this case, it would be the "L" for Lowell.

3. Add the first, third, and fifth numbers in the DEA number together.

   Example: 2 + 5 + 5 = 12.

4. Next add the second, fourth, and sixth numbers together and multiply by 2.

   Example: 4 + 5 + 6 = 15; 15 × 2 = 30

5. Finally, add 12 and 30: 12 + 30 = 42. The last digit "2" should match the last number in the prescriber's DEA number.

The physician's DEA numbers on the practice prescriptions are for practice only and are not actual numbers. To add a doctor to the computer system, refer to the physician list in Appendix C.

ENTERING A NEW PRESCRIPTION

To get started with entering new prescriptions, go to the **Main-1** screen (Figure 8-1) and click on the **Rx-Scrn** button if the screen is not open already.

After you have your prescription and you have read it to verify the information and the medication prescribed, start entering the prescription. In the **Rx Information** box, type an asterisk (*) (Figure 8-2). This will open up all of the boxes in the screen to allow new information to be entered.

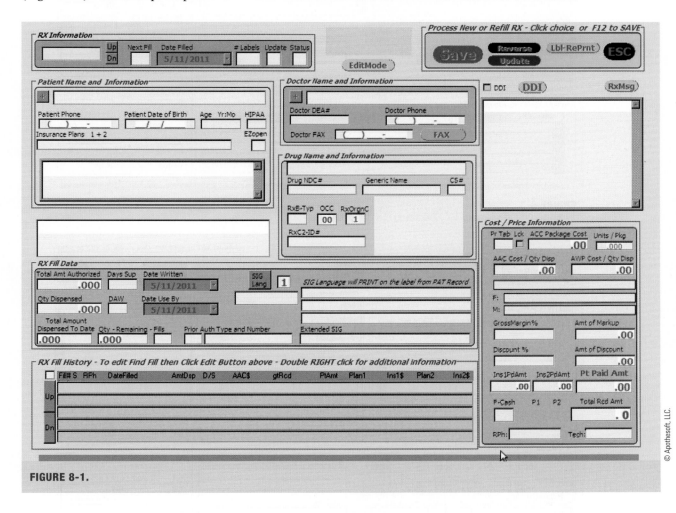

FIGURE 8-1.

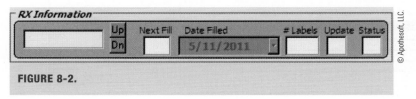

FIGURE 8-2.

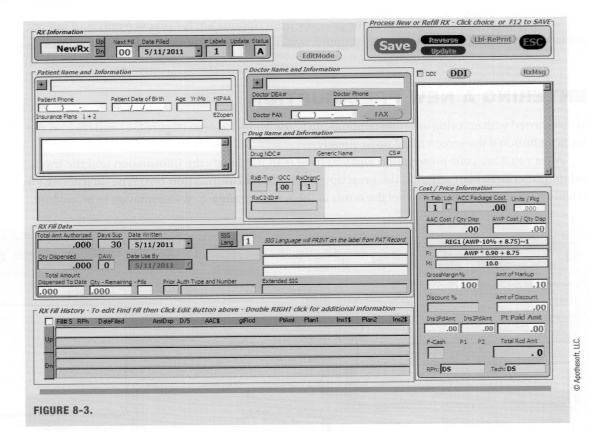

FIGURE 8-3.

© Apothesoft, LLC.

FIGURE 8-4.

© Cengage Learning 2012

After entering the asterisk (*) in the Rx Information box, **NewRx** will appear in the box (Figure 8-3), and the cursor will move to the **Patient Name** and Information box.

To begin, type the patient's name or click on the plus sign (+) that is next to the name to retrieve last patient if you are filling more than one new prescription. If this is a new patient, after you type the name and hit (**ENTER**), the patient screen, **Pt-Scrn** (Figure 8-4), will open, prompting you to enter the patient information. After you have completed the patient information screen, click on **SAVE** and then the **Return Rec** button at top of screen.

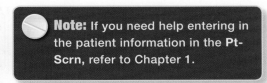

Note: If you need help entering in the patient information in the Pt-Scrn, refer to Chapter 1.

When the **Rx-Scrn** returns, you will notice that some of the information is filled in already. The cursor is now in the **Doctor Name and Information** box (Figure 8-5). Again, if this information is not in the computer system, you will be taken automatically to the **Dr-Scrn** to complete the physician information. The same is true for the **Drug Name and Information** box. If the drug is not in the drug list, you will be taken to the **Dg-Scrn**. Complete the drug information and return to the **Rx-Scrn** (Figure 8-6). And remember to click on **SAVE** button.

After you return to the **Rx-Scrn**, enter the information in the **Rx Fill Data** box. In the **Total Amt Authorized** box, enter the dollar amount

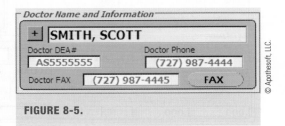

FIGURE 8-5.

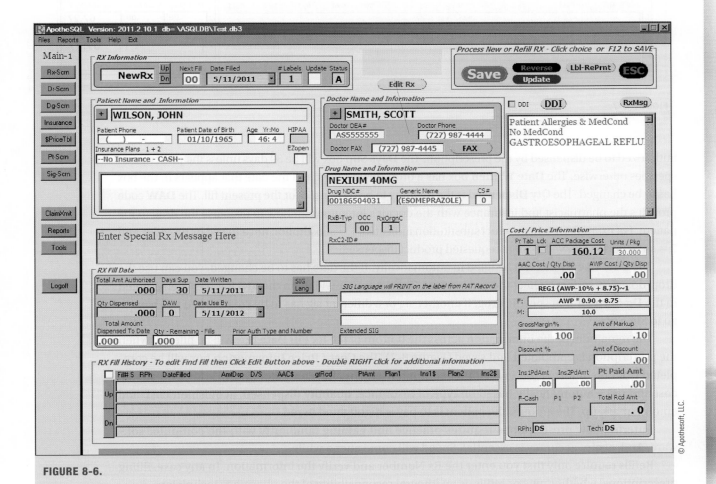

FIGURE 8-6.

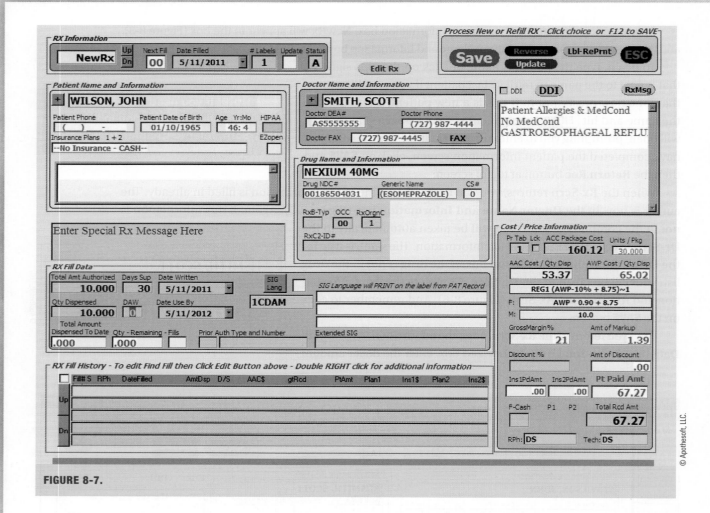

FIGURE 8-7.

© Apothesoft, LLC.

authorized to be dispensed by the prescription. The **Days Sup** box will be 30 days unless the prescription specifies otherwise. The **Date Written** box has a drop-down calendar if the date that appears in the box has to be changed. The **Qty Dispensed** is the quantity to be dispensed for the present fill. The **DAW** code provides the pharmacist and insurance with the doctor's intentions on how to dispense the drug to the patient. For example, 0 = no product substitution indicated, 1 = substitution not allowed by provider, and 2 = substitution allowed–patient requested product dispensed.

The **Date Use By** box will be filled in automatically. If the date has to be changed, you can use the drop-down calendar to select the correct date. The computer will fill in the **SIG** if it has been entered in the **Dg-Scrn** for that specific drug. If another sig or a different sig has to be created, you will have to go to **Sig-Scrn**.

The remainder of the information across the bottom of the **Rx Fill Data** box will be filled in when the prescription is completed and saved (Figure 8-7). The **Cost / Price Information** box will be completed from the information in the other computer screens. The computer system will calculate the cost and price automatically based on type of insurance, quantity dispensed, acquisition cost, and amount mark-up. The amount the patient is to pay is highlighted in red.

Entering new prescriptions requires practice and gaining familiarity with the computer software. And, again, accuracy is essential. Speed will come after a while.

Refills require only that you enter the Rx Number and verify the information. In any case, filling prescriptions, whether new or refills, is an integral responsibility of the pharmacy technician.

EXERCISE I

Enter the following prescriptions. Remember that you may have to enter in the medication and the physician. Refer to Appendix C for additional information.

Scott Smith, M.D.
Internal Medicine Specialist
1234 West Lerner Street
St. Petersburg, Florida 33716
727-555-0123

Patient Name: _Jason Wilson_   Date: _Use current date_

Address: _805 West Sumter Ave_

Rx:

    Nexium 40 mg
        1 cap po QD for GERD
        Disp: 10 (ten)

Substitution Allowed _____   Signature: _Scott Smith_ M.D.

Refills: _____0_____ 1 2 3 4   DEA Number: _AS5555555_

© Cengage Learning 2012

Brian Bonea, M.D.
Rheumatologist
123 Test Street
Test, Wyoming 82000
688-555-0145

Patient Name: _Robin Copper_   Date: _Use current date_

Address: _2145 Right Ave_

Rx:

    Arthrotec 75 mg
        1 tab po BID for RA
        Disp: 60 (sixty)

Substitution Allowed _____   Signature: _Brian Bonea_ M.D.

Refills: _____ 1 ②3 4   DEA Number: _AH5555555_

© Cengage Learning 2012

Thomas Westfield, M.D.
Gastroenterologist
1234 Halfwater Avenue
St. Petersburg, Florida 33716
727-555-0167

Patient Name: *Wanda James*   Date: Use current date

Address: *4010 Coastal Way*

Rx:

Aciphex 20 mg
1 tab po QD after breackfast for ulcers
Disp: 30 (thirty)

Substitution Allowed ___X___   Signature: *Thomas Westfield* ____M.D.

Refills: _____ 1②3 4   DEA Number: BW6666666

© Cengage Learning 2012

Mac U Feelgoud, M.D.
General Surgery
1234 West Lerner Street
St. Petersburg, Florida 33716
727-555-0189

Patient Name: *Roger Horton*   Date: Use current date

Address: *7721 Corbet Ave*

Rx:

Valium 5 mg
2 tabs po 2 hours before procedure
Disp: 2 (two)

Substitution Allowed ___X___   Signature: *Mac Feelgoud* ____M.D.

Refills: _____0_____ 1 2 3 4   DEA Number: AF5555555

© Cengage Learning 2012

Scott Smith, M.D.
Internal Medicine Specialist
1234 West Lerner Street
St. Petersburg, Florida 33716
727-555-0123

Patient Name: *Bonnie Harris*   Date: Use current date

Address: *6610 Woodlawn Street*

Rx:

    Actos 15 mg
        1 tab po QD for diabetes
        Disp: 30 (thirty)

Substitution Allowed _____   Signature: *Scott Smith* _____ M.D.

Refills: _____ 1 (2) 3 4   DEA Number: AS5555555

© Cengage Learning 2012

Joyce White, D.O.
Ophthalmologist
6789 Lester Avenue Suite A
Tampa, Florida 33711
813-555-0176

Patient Name: *Thomas Aspen*   Date: Use current date

Address: *1200 Waters Street*

Rx:

    Restasis
        Instill 1 gtt ou Q12H for dry eyes
        Disp: 1 box (one)

Substitution Allowed _____   Signature: *Joyce White* _____ D.O.

Refills: _____ 1 (2) 3 4   DEA Number: BW1235236

© Cengage Learning 2012

Mac U Feelgoud, M.D.
General Surgery
1234 West Lerner Street
St. Petersburg, Florida 33716
727-555-0189

Patient Name: *Greg Smith*   Date: Use current date

Address: *845 North Iris Ave*

Rx:

Ultracet
    2 tabs po Q4-6H prn for pain
    Disp: 60 (sixty)

Substitution Allowed _____   Signature: *Mac Feelgoud* M.D.

Refills: _____*0*_____ 1 2 3 4   DEA Number: AF5555555

© Cengage Learning 2012

Thomas Westfield, M.D.
Gastroenterologist
1234 Halfwater Avenue
St. Petersburg, Florida 33716
727-555-0167

Patient Name: *Grace Wilson*   Date: Use current date

Address: *520 Grayson Road*

Rx:

Reglan 10 mg
    1 tab po QID 30 minutes AC and HS
    Disp: 120 (one hundred twenty)

Substitution Allowed __*X*__   Signature: *Thomas Westfield* M.D.

Refills: _____ 1 2 (3) 4   DEA Number: BW6666666

© Cengage Learning 2012

Markus Welby, M.D.
General Practitioner
1234 West Lerner Street
St. Petersburg, Florida 33716
688-555-0110

Patient Name: _Sam Turner_____ Date: _Use current date___

Address: _9902 Reader Road_____

Rx:

    Cortisporin-TC OTIC
       5 gtts left ear 3-4 times daily
       Disp: 10 ml (ten)

Substitution Allowed _____   Signature: _Markus Welby_____ M.D.

Refills: _____ 1 ② 3 4   DEA Number: _BB5555555_____

© Cengage Learning 2012

Brian Bonea, M.D.
Rheumatologist
123 Test Street
Test, Wyoming 82000
688-555-0145

Patient Name: _Bill Stevens_____ Date: _Use current date___

Address: _2610 Justin Street_____

Rx:

    Mobic 7.5 mg
       1 tab po QD for joint pain
       Disp: 30 (thirty)

Substitution Allowed __X___   Signature: _Brian Bonea_____ M.D.

Refills: ___6_____ 1 2 3 4   DEA Number: _AH5555555_____

© Cengage Learning 2012

Joyce White, D.O.
Ophthalmologist
6789 Lester Avenue Suite A
Tampa, Florida 33711
813-555-0176

Patient Name: *Rose Winter*   Date: Use current date

Address: *1120 Lakewood Road*

Rx:

Acular
        Instill 1 gtt each eye QID for seasonal conjunctivitis
        Disp: 10 ml (ten)

Substitution Allowed _____   Signature: *Joyce White* _____ D.O.

Refills: _____ 1 ②3 4   DEA Number: BW1235236

© Cengage Learning 2012

Jason Jones, M.D.
Internal Medicine Specialist
469 Medical Circle Suite B
Ocala, Florida 37370
612-555-0137

Patient Name: *Lisa Rough*   Date: Use current date

Address: *1316 Runner Way*

Rx:

Phenergan 12.5 mg
        1 tab po BID for NV
        Disp: 60 (sixty)

Substitution Allowed ___X___   Signature: *Jason Jones* _____ M.D.

Refills: _____ 1 2③4   DEA Number: AJ2346786

© Cengage Learning 2012

Russell Livingston, D.O.
General Medicine
987 Circle Back Way
Tarpon Springs, Florida 33720
727-555-0146

Patient Name: _Bonnie Thompson_   Date: Use current date

Address: _3015 Water Canal Street_

Rx:

     Spiriva
          Inhale QD
          Disp: 1 (one)

Substitution Allowed _____   Signature: _Russell Livingston_ D.O.

Refills: ____6____ 1 2 3 4   DEA Number: _BL6547822_

© Cengage Learning 2012

William Astor, M.D.
Cardiologist
1418 West River Road
Spring Waters, Tennessee 37328
618-555-0155

Patient Name: _George Roberts_   Date: Use current date

Address: _613 Wilkerson Road_

Rx:

     Lopressor 100 mg
          1 tab po BID for CHF
          Disp: 60 (sixty)

Substitution Allowed ___X___   Signature: _William Astor_ M.D.

Refills: _____ ①2 3 4   DEA Number: _AA6352813_

© Cengage Learning 2012

Roger Lowell, M.D.
Orthopedic Surgeon
8020 University Circle
Grandview, Alabama 32716
606-555-0109

Patient Name: _Ted Kline_____ Date: _Use current date___

Address: _9090 College Lane_____

Rx:

    Vicoprofen
        1 tab po Q 4-6 H prn for post op pain
        Disp: 30 (thirty)

Substitution Allowed _____   Signature: _Roger Lowell_____ M.D.

Refills: _____0_____ 1 2 3 4   DEA Number: _BL9562125_____

© Cengage Learning 2012

Jane Wester, M.D.
Gerontology
8080 West Lane, Suite A
St. Petersburg, Florida 33716
727-555-0113

Patient Name: _Chester Thompson_____ Date: _Use current date___

Address: _5858 Brookstone Road_____

Rx:

    Razadyne 4 mg
        1 tab po with AM & PM meals for moderate Alzheimers
        Disp: 60 (sixty)

Substitution Allowed _____   Signature: _Jane Wester_____ M.D.

Refills: _____0_____ 1 2 3 4   DEA Number: _BW8541238_____

© Cengage Learning 2012

Jason Jones, M.D.
Internal Medicine Specialist
469 Medical Circle Suite B
Ocala, Florida 37370
612-555-0137

Patient Name: _Mike Fortuna_   Date: _Use current date_

Address: _8080 Tall Oaks Road_

Rx:

    Luvox CR 100 mg
        1 cap po qHS for OCD
        Disp: 30 (thirty)

Substitution Allowed _____   Signature: _Jason Jones_ M.D.

Refills: _____ ①2 3 4   DEA Number: _AJ2346786_

© Cengage Learning 2012

Russell Livingston, D.O.
General Medicine
987 Circle Back Way
Tarpon Springs, Florida 33720
727-555-0146

Patient Name: _Ken Summer_   Date: _Use current date_

Address: _765 Watson Road_

Rx:

    Arthrotec 75 mg
        1 tab BID for OA pain
        Disp: 60 (sixty)

Substitution Allowed _____   Signature: _Russell Livingston_ D.O.

Refills: _____ 1 2③4   DEA Number: _BL6547822_

© Cengage Learning 2012

William Astor, M.D.
Cardiologist
1418 West River Road
Spring Waters, Tennessee 37328
618-555-0155

Patient Name: _Traci Farmer_____   Date:_Use current date___

Address: __771 River Run Road_____

Rx:

    400 mg Trental
       1 tab po TID with food for intermittent claudication
       Disp: 90 (ninety)

Substitution Allowed _____   Signature: _William Astor_____M.D.

Refills: _____7_____ 1 2 3 4   DEA Number: _AA6352813_____

© Cengage Learning 2012

Roger Lowell, M.D.
Orthopedic Surgeon
8020 University Circle
Grandview, Alabama 32716
606-555-0109

Patient Name: _Joe Wilson_____   Date:_Use current date___

Address: _4050 Technology Way_____

Rx:

    Percocet 5/325
       1-2 tabs Q 6 Hrs prn for post op pain
       Disp: 50 (fifty)

Substitution Allowed _X___   Signature: _Roger Lowell_____M.D.

Refills: _____0_____ 1 2 3 4   DEA Number: _BL9562125_____

© Cengage Learning 2012

James Campbell, M.D.
Pediatrician
9080 Turner Street
Hollywood, Florida 33896
804-555-0122

Patient Name: _Kim Sands_   Date: _Use current date_

Address: _4540 Kindle Lane_

Rx:

　　Floxin Otic 0.3%
　　　　Instill 5 gtts in affected ear BID for 10 days for otitis media
　　　　Disp: 10 ml (ten)

Substitution Allowed ___X___   Signature: _James Campbell_ M.D.

Refills: ___0___ 1 2 3 4   DEA Number: _AC5641234_

© Cengage Learning 2012

Kathy O'Conner, D.O.
Internal Medicine Specialist
2345 Miller Road Way
St. Petersburg, Florida 33716
727-555-0144

Patient Name: _Mary Solvin_   Date: _Use current date_

Address: _5828 49th Street_

Rx:

　　Maxalt 5 mg
　　　　1 tab po at onset of HA, may repeat in 2 HRS if no relief (not to
　　　　exceed 3 per day)
　　　　Disp: 6 (six)

Substitution Allowed _____   Signature: _Kathy O'Connor_ D.O.

Refills: ___6___ 1 2 3 4   DEA Number: _AO8976326_

© Cengage Learning 2012

William Astor, M.D.
Cardiologist
1418 West River Road
Spring Waters, Tennessee 37328
618-555-0155

Patient Name: _Selina Wright_   Date: Use current date

Address: _2625 Throughbred Street_

Rx:

    Tambocor 100 mg
        1 po Q12H for arrhythmias
        Disp: 60 (sixty)

Substitution Allowed ___X___   Signature: _William Astor_ M.D.

Refills: ___12___ 1 2 3 4   DEA Number: _AA6352813_

© Cengage Learning 2012

Markus Welby, M.D.
General Practitioner
1234 West Lerner Street
St. Petersburg, Florida 33716
688-555-0110

Patient Name: _Mary Taylor_   Date: Use current date

Address: _9012 Intercoastal Way_

Rx:

    Repliva 21/7
        1 tab po QD for 28 days for iron deficiency anemia
        Disp: 1 pak (one)

Substitution Allowed _____   Signature: _Markus Welby_ M.D.

Refills: ___0___ 1 2 3 4   DEA Number: _BB5555555_

© Cengage Learning 2012

Scott Smith, M.D.
Internal Medicine Specialist
1234 West Lerner Street
St. Petersburg, Florida 33716
727-555-0123

Patient Name: _Tommy Klein_____   Date: _Use current date____

Address: _652 Bayway Drive_____

Rx:

    Lovaza 4 gm
       1 cap po QD for elevated triglycerides
       Disp: 30 (thirty)

Substitution Allowed _____   Signature: _Scott Smith_____ M.D.

Refills: _____ 1 ②3 4   DEA Number: _AS5555555_____

© Cengage Learning 2012

Jane Wester, M.D.
Gerontology
8080 West Lane, Suite A
St. Petersburg, Florida 33716
727-555-0113

Patient Name: _Arnold Winston_____   Date: _Use current date____

Address: _1020 Turner Street_____

Rx:

    DDAVP Nasal Spray 10 mcg
       Instill 1 spray internasally q HS
       Disp: 1 (one)

Substitution Allowed _____   Signature: _Jane Wester_____ M.D.

Refills: _____ 1 2 3④   DEA Number: _BW8541238_____

© Cengage Learning 2012

Roger Lowell, M.D.
Orthopedic Surgeon
8020 University Circle
Grandview, Alabama 32716
606-555-0109

Patient Name: _Tammy Speed_ Date: Use current date

Address: _1813 History Circle_

Rx:

    Spectracef 200 mg
       1 tb po BID X10 days for infection
       Disp: 20 (twenty)

Substitution Allowed _____ Signature: _Roger Lowell_ M.D.

Refills: _____0_____ 1 2 3 4 DEA Number: _BL9562125_

© Cengage Learning 2012

Kathy O'Conner, D.O.
Internal Medicine Specialist
2345 Miller Road Way
St. Petersburg, Florida 33716
727-555-0144

Patient Name: _William Johnson_ Date: Use current date

Address: _4602 Coral Beach Drive_

Rx:

    Adovart 0.5 mg
       1 cap po QD for BPH
       Disp: 30 (thirty)

Substitution Allowed _____ Signature: _Kathy O'Connor_ D.O.

Refills: _____ 1 2 ③ 4 DEA Number: _AO8976326_

© Cengage Learning 2012

James Campbell, M.D.
Pediatrician
9080 Turner Street
Hollywood, Florida 33896
804-555-0122

Patient Name: _Karla Watts_   Date: _Use current date_

Address: _192 Aspen Trail_

Rx:

    Duratuss AC 12
       5 ml po Q 12 H for congestion
       Disp: 60 ml (sixty)

Substitution Allowed _____   Signature: _James Campbell_ M.D.

Refills: ___0___ 1 2 3 4   DEA Number: _AC5641234_

© Cengage Learning 2012

Markus Welby, M.D.
General Practitioner
1234 West Lerner Street
St. Petersburg, Florida 33716
688-555-0110

Patient Name: _Susan Turner_   Date: _Use current date_

Address: _8855 Corvette Ave Apt 10_

Rx:

    Crestor 5 mg
       1 tab po QD for elevated cholesterol
       Disp: 30 (thirty)

Substitution Allowed _____   Signature: _Markus Welby_ M.D.

Refills: ___0___ 1 2 3 4   DEA Number: _BB5555555_

© Cengage Learning 2012

CRITICAL THINKING

1. Discuss the importance of having the patient's medical history in the computer system when a filling a prescription.

2. Why do you have to verify the prescribing physician's DEA number?

3. What action would you take if the requested medication is not in the computer system?

4. When receiving a prescription for a schedule drug, would you check the number of refills requested before filling the prescription?

5. Why is the patient's correct birth date necessary?

6. Why is the correct days supply necessary when entering a prescription?

7. For what reasons should the pharmacy technician maintain good communication with the pharmacist?

8. Why should the pharmacy technician be able to multi-task?

9. Why is attention to detail an essential trait for a pharmacy technician?

10. What would you do if you were to discover a mistake in a prescription?

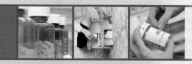

CHAPTER 9

Running Reports

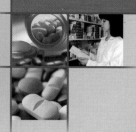

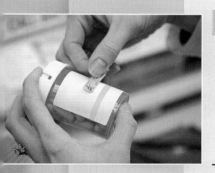

LEARNING OBJECTIVES

1. Discuss the information needed to run daily reports.

2. Explain the information contained in the sales reports.

3. Point out the importance of the drug profile report.

4. Explain why the patient billing report may be given to the patient.

5. Discuss the importance of the patient profile report.

A pharmacy must have access to a myriad of reports to track sales, inventory, and patient drug profiles. Federal and state guidelines require many different reports, and the pharmacy must be able to produce them in hardcopy during an inspection. The task of running daily reports may be one of the pharmacy technician's job responsibilities. This chapter covers many of the reports available and how to pull these reports from the pharmacy software program.

Running reports represents a valuable tool for managing the pharmacy, and reports also must be run and kept on file for legal purposes. This program, like all programs, provides the capability to run such reports. If the pharmacy has a specific need for a customized report, the software supplier can write a program to fill that need.

As a pharmacy technician, you may be assigned the task of running daily sales reports and daily sales reports of controlled substances. Also, if you are working with the pharmacist to maintain pharmacy records, you may be asked to run other reports periodically and maintain them in files. The type of pharmacy reports you may work with depends on the pharmacy setting in which you are working and your level of responsibility or job description.

To begin, access the reports function either by clicking on **Reports** at the top of the screen in the task bar or by clicking on the **Reports** button on the left side of the screen (Figure 9-1).

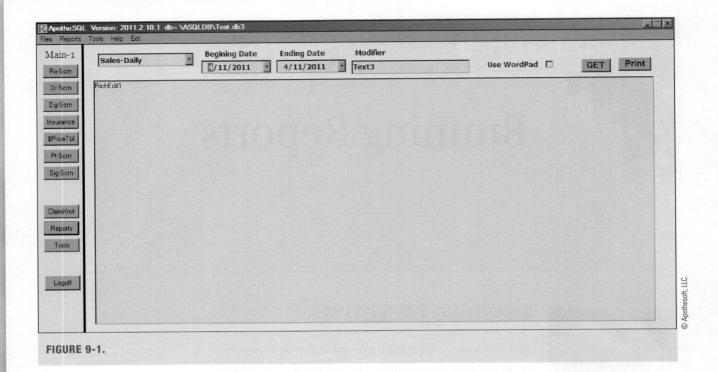

© Apothesoft, LLC.

FIGURE 9-1.

THE SALES REPORT

The sales report allows the pharmacy to keep track of how many prescriptions were filled on any given day. This report lists the total number of prescriptions and lists each prescription, showing the prescription number, patient, physician, drug, and quantity, NDC number, and sig code. It also indicates whether the prescription was or was not a controlled substance. If the prescription is a controlled substance, the schedule number will be listed.

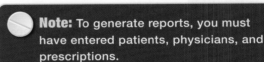

Note: To generate reports, you must have entered patients, physicians, and prescriptions.

Accounting information is one of the most important pieces of information for the pharmacy owner or operations pharmacist. The sales report provides a breakdown of the cost of acquisition for the amount of drug dispensed, how much the patient paid, how much the insurance provider paid, and which insurance plan covered the prescription.

The report totals all prescriptions within a specified time period and in addition gives the amount of profit and margin percentage on all prescriptions. All compounds that were sold will be broken out separately in the report. By providing sales information on a daily, weekly, and monthly basis, the pharmacy is able to determine how the acquisition cost relates to the gross sales and profit margin.

Running the Daily Sales Report

To start running the report, select **Reports** on the task bar at the top of the screen or by clicking on the **Reports** button on the left side of the screen. The screen will open to a blank screen with **Sales-Daily** showing in the drop-down box. At the top of the screen, to the right of the drop down box, are two boxes for entering a date range for the report. The desired **Beginning Date** and **Ending Date** can be entered in the boxes. If you have to use the calendar function, simply click on the down arrow in either box and select the beginning and ending date range for the report (Figure 9-2).

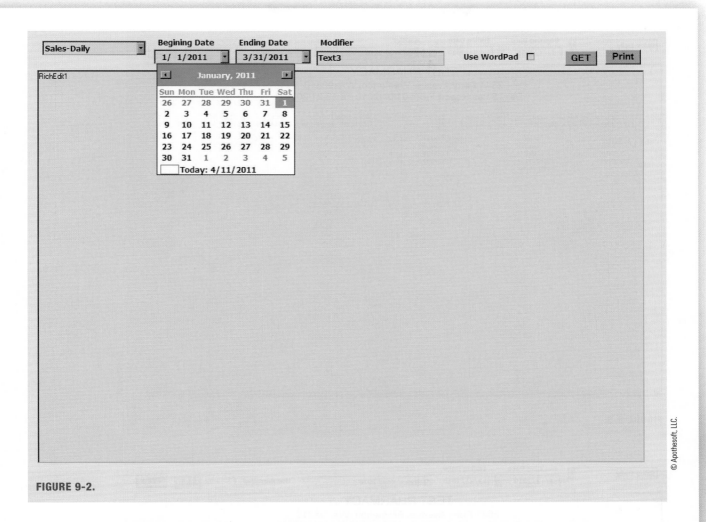

FIGURE 9-2.

After entering the desired date range, move to the **GET** button on the same line to the right and click on it. The **Daily Sales Report** covering the requested dates will appear (Figure 9-3). Not all of the information contained in the report shows up on the screen. Across the bottom of the screen is a bar that, if clicked on and pulled to the right, will show the rest of the report.

To print the report, simply click on the **Print** button and the **Print Setup** box will pop up. If the default printer does not have to be changed, click on **OK** and the report will print on the default printer (Figure 9-4). If the report has to print in the landscape format, click on the Landscape button before printing.

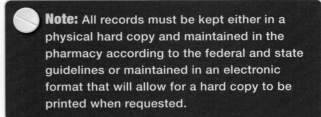

Note: All records must be kept either in a physical hard copy and maintained in the pharmacy according to the federal and state guidelines or maintained in an electronic format that will allow for a hard copy to be printed when requested.

RUNNING THE DAILY-SALES CS REPORT

The **Daily-Sales CS** report is the second report listed in the drop-down box in the Reports screen. This report lists all sales of controlled substances. The report contains the same information as the **Daily Sales Report** but lists only the controlled substances (Figure 9-5). The controlled substances sales reports are maintained in a separate file. Just as with the daily sales reports, the controlled substances sales reports can be maintained in an electronic file but must be able to produce a hard copy when requested by an inspecting agency.

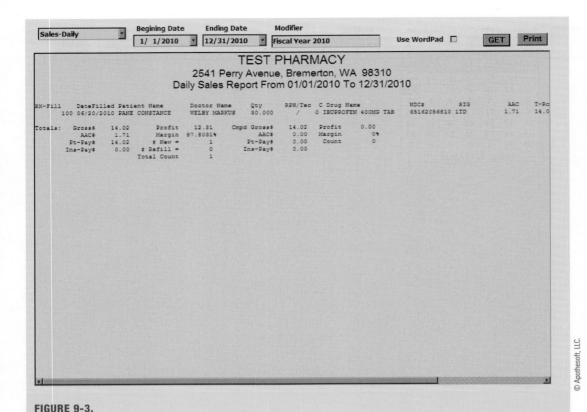

FIGURE 9-3.

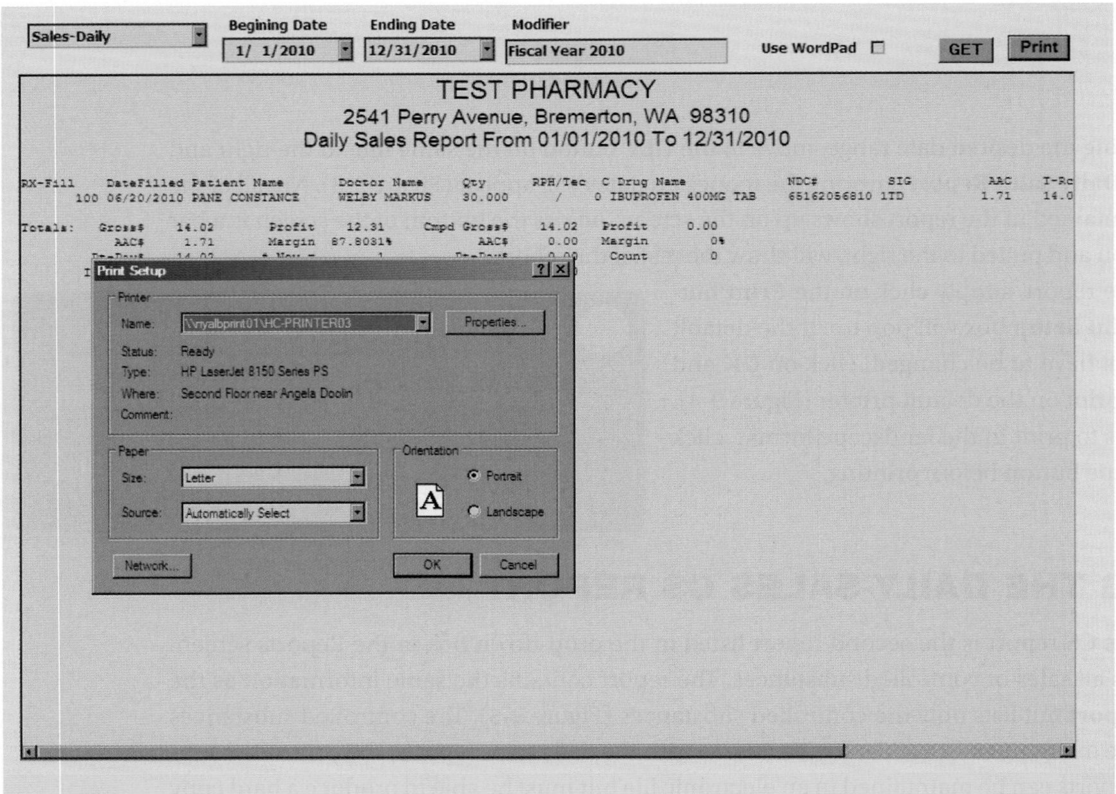

FIGURE 9-4.

© Apothesoft, LLC.

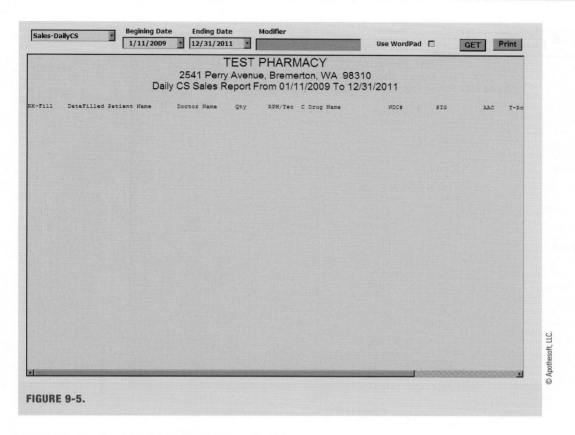

FIGURE 9-5.

Running the Sales-Statistics Report

As with the other sales reports, the **Sales-Statistics** report shows the number of prescriptions sold during a designated time frame, dollar sales, acquisition cost, net profit, and margin percentage in four different categories. The **Sales-Statistics** report breaks down the sales by **CASH**, **WELFARE**, and **THIRD PARTY** sales. The report also breaks out the compounds sales from the above totals and shows the total compound sales at the bottom of the report page (Figure 9-6).

The **Sales-Statistics** report is used to review the overall sales activity. It does not show the patient, physician, or prescription information. The pharmacy manager can use this report for a quick analysis of all sales.

Running the Sales-By-InsPlan Report

Once the report has been selected from the drop-down list, enter the date range for which you want to analyze insurance sales. In the **Modifier** box, enter the insurance plan number you want to review. The **Sales-By InsPlan** report will show the same information as the **Sales-Daily** report but is limited to only the insurance plan listed in the modifier box (Figure 9-7).

RUNNING THE DRUG UTILIZATION REPORT

The **DrugUtilization** report has a preset formula in the **Modifier** box to pull and list all drugs dispensed for the designated period of time and the quantity of each drug (Figure 9-8). This is an excellent report for the pharmacy purchaser/buyer to use for ordering drugs to maintain a maximum quantity on the shelves.

 Note: The screen shown in Figure 9-7 does not contain information for the insurance plan because the claim was not processed.

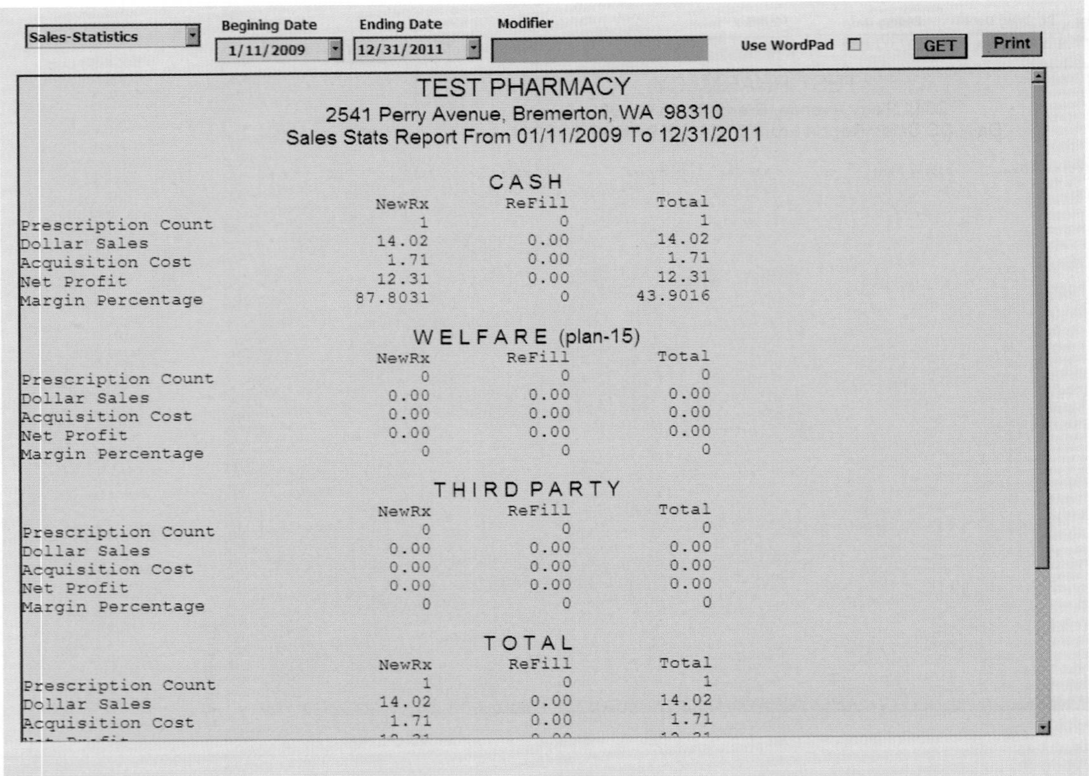

| Sales-Statistics ▼ | Begining Date 1/11/2009 ▼ | Ending Date 12/31/2011 ▼ | Modifier | | Use WordPad ☐ | GET | Print |

```
                    TEST PHARMACY
          2541 Perry Avenue, Bremerton, WA  98310
        Sales Stats Report From 01/11/2009 To 12/31/2011

                         CASH
                    NewRx      ReFill         Total
Prescription Count    1          0             1
Dollar Sales         14.02      0.00          14.02
Acquisition Cost      1.71      0.00           1.71
Net Profit           12.31      0.00          12.31
Margin Percentage    87.8031    0             43.9016

                   WELFARE (plan-15)
                    NewRx      ReFill         Total
Prescription Count    0          0             0
Dollar Sales         0.00       0.00          0.00
Acquisition Cost     0.00       0.00          0.00
Net Profit           0.00       0.00          0.00
Margin Percentage    0          0             0

                    THIRD PARTY
                    NewRx      ReFill         Total
Prescription Count    0          0             0
Dollar Sales         0.00       0.00          0.00
Acquisition Cost     0.00       0.00          0.00
Net Profit           0.00       0.00          0.00
Margin Percentage    0          0             0

                       TOTAL
                    NewRx      ReFill         Total
Prescription Count    1          0             1
Dollar Sales         14.02      0.00          14.02
Acquisition Cost      1.71      0.00           1.71
```

© Apothesoft, LLC.

FIGURE 9-6.

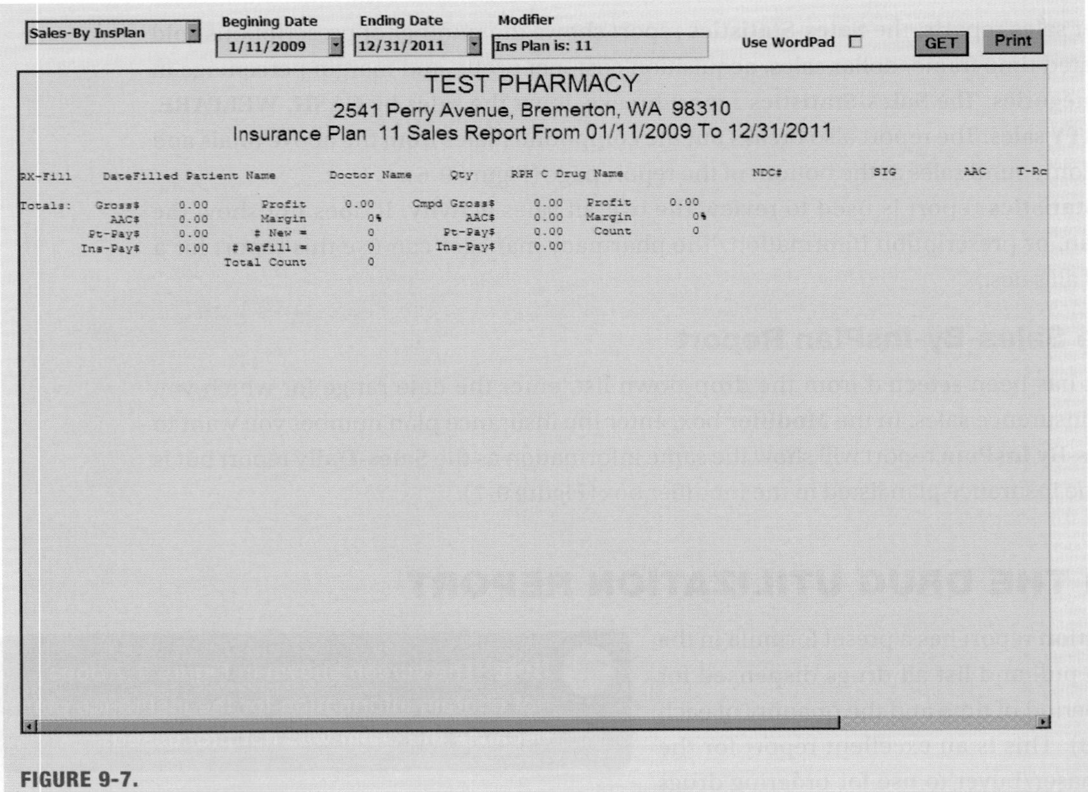

| Sales-By InsPlan ▼ | Begining Date 1/11/2009 ▼ | Ending Date 12/31/2011 ▼ | Modifier Ins Plan is: 11 | | Use WordPad ☐ | GET | Print |

```
                         TEST PHARMACY
               2541 Perry Avenue, Bremerton, WA  98310
      Insurance Plan  11 Sales Report From 01/11/2009 To 12/31/2011

RX-Fill   DateFilled Patient Name   Doctor Name   Qty  RPH C Drug Name           NDC#        SIG      AAC   T-Rc

Totals:  Gross$  0.00    Profit    0.00   Cmpd Gross$  0.00   Profit   0.00
         AAC$    0.00    Margin    0%              AAC$  0.00   Margin   0%
         Pt-Pay$ 0.00    # New =   0           Pt-Pay$  0.00   Count    0
         Ins-Pay$ 0.00   # Refill = 0          Ins-Pay$ 0.00
                         Total Count 0
```

© Apothesoft, LLC.

FIGURE 9-7.

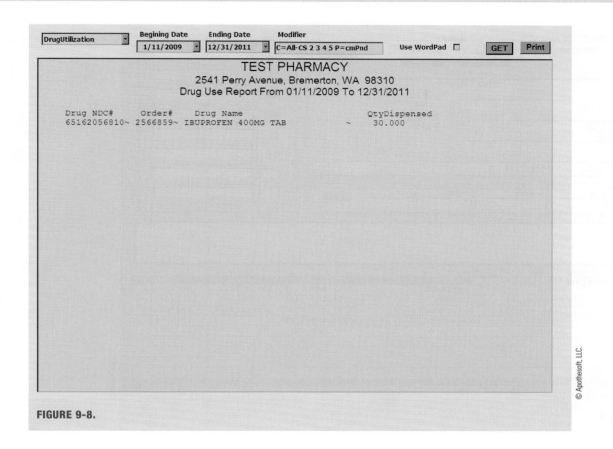

FIGURE 9-8.

RUNNING THE PROFILE BY DOCTOR REPORT

To run the **Profile-For Dr** report, first select the physician by clicking on the **Dr-Scrn** button. Then select the physician for which the report is to be run (Figure 9-9).

When you select the time period for the report, the desired physician's name should appear in the **Modifier** box. Click on the **GET** box, and the information will appear (Figure 9-10). The report provides a list of all prescriptions filled for patients under this provider's name. In addition, a summary of the gross amount of sales and profits from this list of prescriptions is part of the report. The report also provides the pharmacist more detailed information on what medications a specific provider is prescribing.

RUNNING THE DRUG PROFILE REPORT

Before running the **Profile-For Dg** report, you must select the drug you want to profile. To start, select the drug by clicking on the **Dg-Scrn** button on the left side of the screen, and then scroll through the **Drug Name * Search List** until you find the desired drug. Make sure that the drug is highlighted in red in the list (Figure 9-11).

Click on the **Reports** button on the left side of the screen, then select the **Profile-For Dg** report from the drop-down screen. After you select the desired date range, the drug you want to profile should appear in the **Modifier** box. After verifying the information, click on the **GET** button. The report will appear for the selected drug (Figure 9-12). This report shows how many times that drug was filled by date, pharmacist, how paid for, how much paid, and quantity dispensed, along with

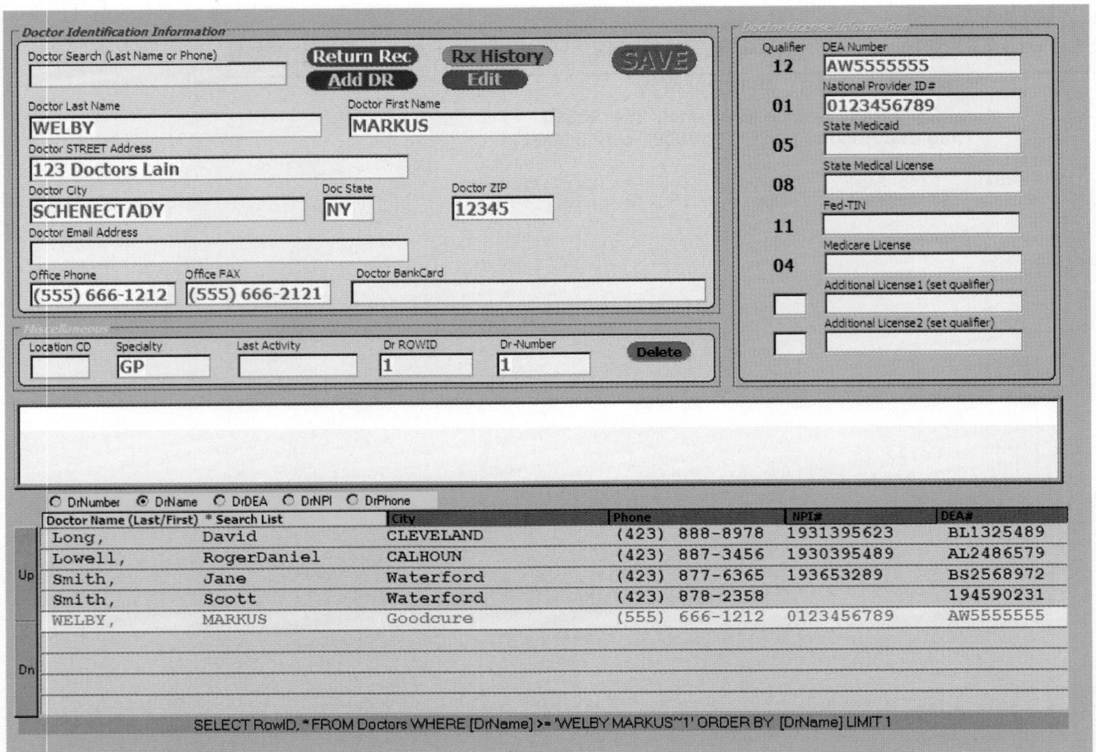

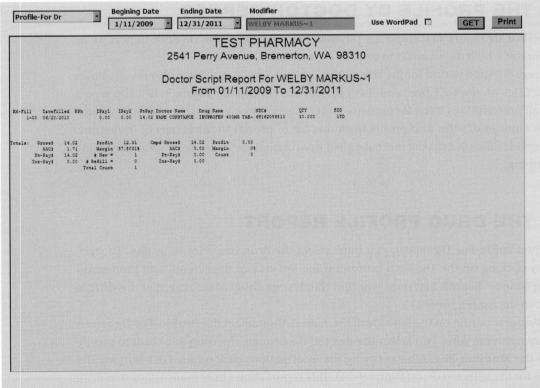

FIGURE 9-9.

FIGURE 9-10.

© Apothesoft, LLC.

© Apothesoft, LLC.

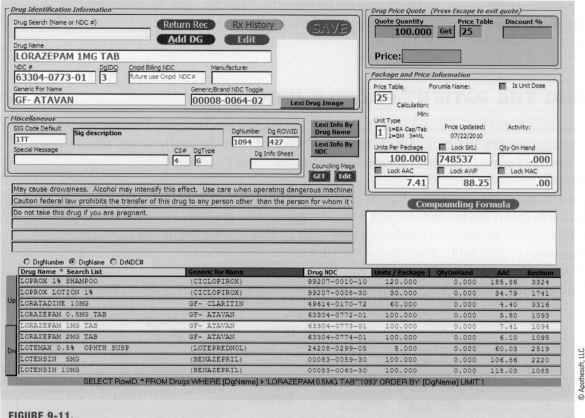

FIGURE 9-11.

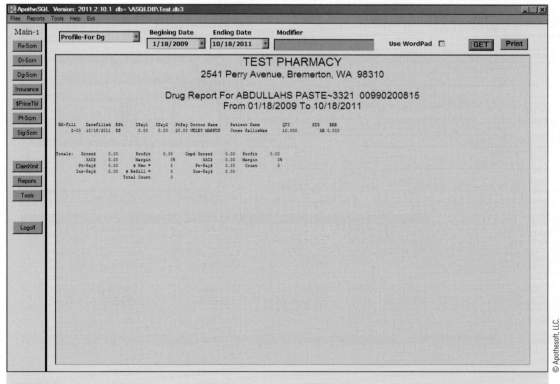

FIGURE 9-12.

© Apothesoft, LLC.

the doctor's name and the patient's name. By printing a report for a specific drug, the pharmacist can review the frequency-of-use patterns and prescribing by an individual provider. The report also contains a breakdown of costs and profits.

RUNNING THE PATIENT PROFILE REPORT

To pull up the **Profile-For Pt** report, the same as for other reports, you first must select the patient screen by clicking on the **Pt-Scrn** button on the left side of the screen. From the patient screen, select the patient from the **Patient Name Search List** (Figure 9-13). Make sure that the patient you wish to find is highlighted.

Next click on the **Reports** button on the left side of the screen. From the drop-down list, select the **Profile-For Pt** report and the patient's name should appear in the **Modifier** box. Before clicking on the **GET** button, be sure that the desired date range is shown in the **Beginning Date** and **Ending Date** boxes (Figure 9-14). After clicking the **GET** button, you will see the report showing the prescription information for that patient. This report allows for the pharmacist's complete review of the patient's medications. In addition, patients can show the report to their primary physician.

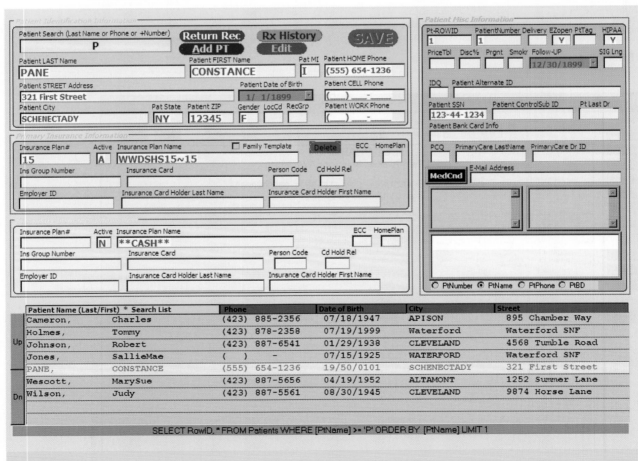

FIGURE 9-13.

© Apothesoft, LLC.

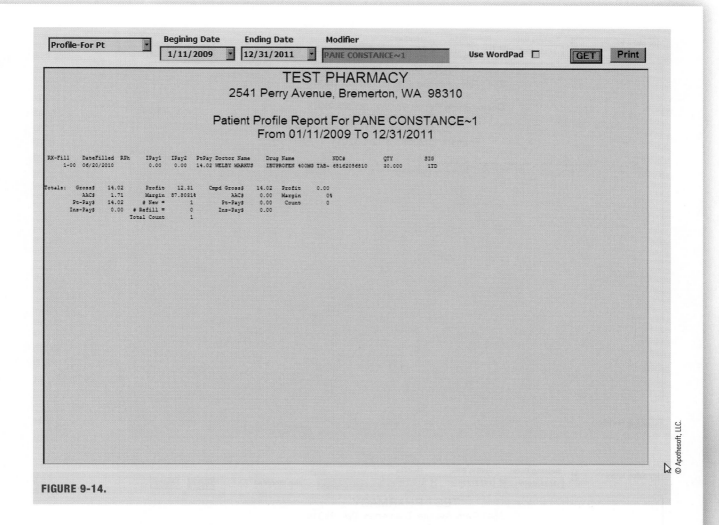

FIGURE 9-14.

RUNNING THE DOCTOR AND PATIENT BILLING REPORTS

As with the **Profile-For Dr** and **Profile-For Pt** reports, you first must select the doctor or patient on whom you wish to run a report. The **Dr Billing Report** and **Pt Billing Report** are selected from the **Reports** screen the same as the other reports. Again, be sure that the date range is correct, along with the **Modifier** box, which contains the correct doctor or patient name, depending on the report.

The **Dr Billing Report** lists the same information as the doctor profile report except that it provides a total cost of all prescriptions written by the provider and a pharmacist signature line for the pharmacist to sign off on the information (Figure 9-15).

The **Pt Billing Report**, like the **Dr Billing Report**, is the same as the patient profile report except that the billing report provides a total amount spent by patients for their prescriptions and a line for a signature of the pharmacist, verifying the information (Figure 9-16). This report may be provided to the patient to use for insurance claims or income taxes.

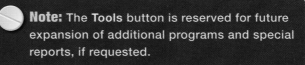

Note: The **Tools** button is reserved for future expansion of additional programs and special reports, if requested.

Reports are valuable tools in managing the pharmacy. They are used by the pharmacist or the pharmacy technician to track expenditures, profit margins, inventory, patient medication

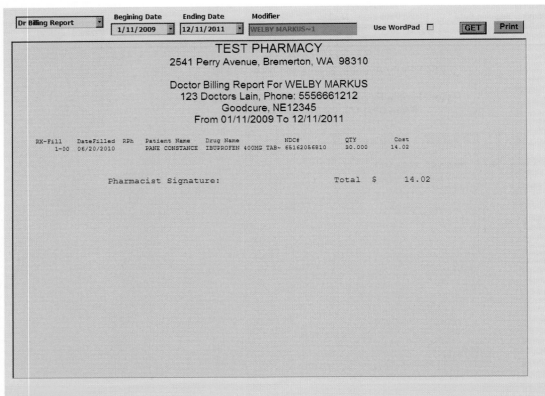

FIGURE 9-15.

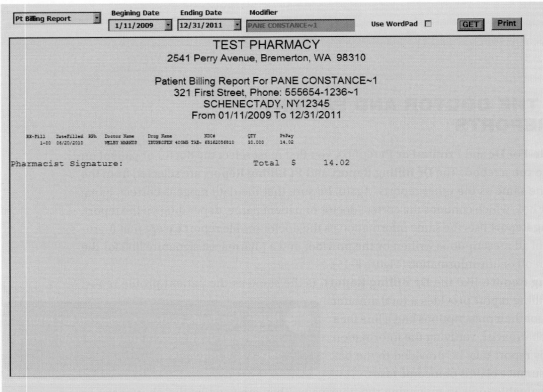

FIGURE 9-16.

utilization, provider prescribing, and payer activity. Computer software providers all develop these reports to assist pharmacy managers in managing the day-to-day operations and to meet federal and state requirements for reporting.

EXERCISE I

Run a **Sales-Daily** report. Review the information for the class of drug and the quantity filled for each class of drug. Also, review the report to make sure that all of the information is complete.

EXERCISE II

Run a **Drug Utilization** report. How would you use this report if you were the pharmacy purchaser/buyer?

EXERCISE III

Run a **Sales-Daily CS Report**. What information can you gain from this report? What classes of drugs would appear on this report? How often should you run this report?

EXERCISE IV

Run a **Sales-Daily** report. What information does this report provide? How often should you run this report? What information is contained on this report that can aid the pharmacy manager in improving the monetary outcome of all sales?

EXERCISE V

If the pharmacist asks for a report that shows only the prescription count and the dollar sales, which report should you run? Run this report.

CRITICAL THINKING

1. If you have to know how much of a specific drug has been dispensed over a defined period of time, what report would you use? Why?

2. If you were placed in charge of doing the inventory for the month, what report would be useful for checking how much of each drug was dispensed during the month?

3. You are asked to verify the count for the controlled substances 3 through 5 dispensed for the day against the perpetual count records. What report would you run to compare with the count records?

4. You receive a call from a patient who wants to know what medications he has had filled at the pharmacy for the last year. What report would you consider running?

5. At the end of the day, you need to know how many prescriptions were filled and the day's gross sales. What report would best provide this information?

6. Which report would you print to provide a total of compound prescriptions filled and the net profit for a week?

7. Some cases request that a physician's prescription activity be made available. Which report do you think would be the best report to run?

8. If you are asked to research the historical use of a specific drug, what report would you select? What information would the report provide?

9. You have been requested to find the margin percentage total for a certain doctor for a given time frame. Which report would you run?

10. You have been asked to find out how much of a specific drug was dispensed for the last week. Which report would you run?

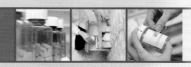

CHAPTER **10**

Medication Administration Records

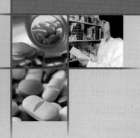

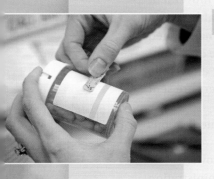

LEARNING OBJECTIVES

1. Indicate who is responsible for managing the medication administration records in the hospital.

2. Discuss the different forms used in a long-term care pharmacy.

3. Point out who verifies the medication and treatment records in the long-term care pharmacy.

4. Discuss the different types of treatment records that may be used during the patient's care.

5. Describe the process of changing the type of records in the hospital.

Depending on the type of pharmacy practice setting, the pharmacy technician may have to deal with several different forms necessary for managing the patient's medications and treatments. Administration of the patient's medications is an issue of compliance, and to ensure that they are done properly, legal documents are required to verify their administration. These records, used by several different healthcare professionals, must be correct. Maintaining the records in the pharmacy is the responsibility of the pharmacy technician. This chapter identifies some of these forms and their uses.

Medication administration records (MARs) constitute one of the reports that a pharmacy technician in a long-term care (LTC) pharmacy may be responsible for maintaining and printing on a monthly basis. Pharmacy technicians in long-term care pharmacies also will be responsible for the physician orders (POs) and treatment administration records (TARs). The pharmacy technician may work in a separate medical records department, depending on the size of the facility.

In hospitals or other large institutions, the medical records are managed by medical records and health information technicians who also may be medical coders or coding specialists. They also may specialize and become cancer registrars. The medication orders are filled by the pharmacist and pharmacy technician within the institution. All departments within an institution channel information to the medical records department.

Within the LTC or Assisted Living Facility (ALF), the MAR serves as a legal record of the medications to be administered to a patient at the facility by a nurse or other health care professional. The medications are taken from the physician orders, which are reviewed and verified by the registered nurse (RN) and then signed by the treating physician. The individual administering the medication to the patient must sign off on the record at the time the medication is administered or a device is applied. The MAR also verifies that appropriate therapy has been provided to the patient. At some facilities, this is referred to as a drug chart.

Prior to the final printing of records for delivery to the facility, there usually is what has been called a "white paper run." The pharmacist views this print-out for correctness and clinical effectiveness of the medication therapy and treatments.

The LTC and ALF facilities and pharmacies use a wide variety of MARs. There is a movement toward what is called an electronic medication record (EMR) or an electronic health record (EHR) in many hospitals, nursing home facilities, and physician offices. The EMR is maintained on the computer instead of in a chart. In large hospitals, the EMR or EHR is accessible on a computer mounted to the medication cart or located next to the patient's bedside. This allows the treating physician to review the record and write new orders electronically. The orders are sent to the appropriate pharmacy or department depending upon the patient's location.

The retail pharmacy also maintains a health record electronically. It lists patients' medications and, if known, their allergies and medical condition.

The common types of pharmacy information that may appear on an MAR are as follows:

- medication: name, dosage strength, route of administration, frequency of administration and times to be administered, indication for use of medication
- diagnosis
- prescribing physician details
- patient information: room and bed number, date of birth
- allergies
- a month chart by days for the nurses/health professionals administering medications to initial when medications were administered.

The back of the MAR will contain nurse's medication notes for recording responses and results of the medication. Also, there will be a chart for blood pressure, temperature, and pulse.

The MAR may be printed in multiple pages or sections. The routine medications will appear first, followed by the as needed or as necessary (PRN) medications. In addition, if the patient is receiving treatments such as wound therapy, there may be an additional printed form, called a treatment administration record (TAR). The TAR is used in the same way as the MAR, but it lists only the treatments the patient is receiving.

In addition are administration records that are used for nutritional supplements administered through the digestive tract (enteral orders) and bladder catheters (catheter orders). These also require the nurse or healthcare professional to sign off on the type of action taken. The enteral orders show how much nutrition was given, how many calories, tube and head-of-bed placement, and type of flushes used. The catheter orders show size of catheter, when to change it, and how it was irrigated.

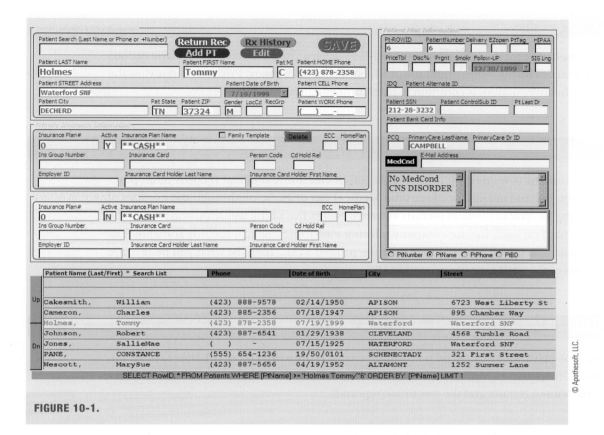

FIGURE 10-1.

Many different pharmacy software systems are used in the different pharmacy practice settings, but they all have the same basic information pertaining to the patient's medications, and all require the nurse or health care professional to sign or initial when the medication, treatment, or feeding is administered.

In the ApotheSoft software program, the information appearing in the patient screen (**Pt-Scrn**) (Figure 10-1) and the drug screen (**Dg-Scrn**) will provide the information to fill the required portions of the MAR.

In the patient screen is a **PtTag** box (Figure 10-2) in the *Patient Misc Information* block. This tag represents a facility or floor where the patient is residing. This **PtTag** is generated by the pharmacy and will consist of any combination of letters to represent a tag attached to the facility name.

Examples of MARs appear in Appendix D. Look at how they can differ. Also, a **Physician Order** sheet is included, which will contain the orders written by the patient's physician. This information is entered into the pharmacy system and is printed on all the other records mentioned above when maintained by a long-term care pharmacy.

> **Note:** The patient medication administration report (MAR) is not available in the demo version of the ApotheSoft program.

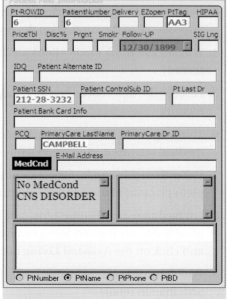

FIGURE 10-2.

EXERCISE I

Go online to the web page for the form suppliers Med-Pass at *www.med-pass.com*. Look at the various types of medical record forms found under the products tab for **Pharmacy**. Print out and review the records, noting what information is common to each form and how they differ.

EXERCISE II

The federal government is requesting implementation of electronic medical records in all practice settings. Go online and search for **Electronic Medical Records**. Scroll through the number of companies offering electronic medical records software. Select five of the websites, and look at the information provided on each for the company offering electronic medical records software. List what you believe are the advantages of EMRs over the printed MAR. Then list what you believe are the disadvantages of the EMR over the printed MAR.

EXERCISE III

Go online and look up various articles on medication errors. Write a brief report on how medication errors may occur in relation to MARs or TARs. Do you think the same number of medication errors can occur using printed reports and the electronic reports?

CRITICAL THINKING

1. Discuss the importance of the medication administration records.
2. Why does the pharmacy technician have to understand how the various records are used during the care of a patient?
3. Look at the back of the various records in the Med-Pass website, *www.med-pass.com*, and discuss the importance of the content on the reverse side of the records.
4. Why do you think medications are separated into Routine and PRN on the medication administration record?
5. Discuss the differences between the various records and how the pharmacy information is used on these records.
6. Thinking about the various pharmacy practice settings, which of the pharmacy practices would be providing medical records and additional information to support medical care?
7. Other than printing forms containing information about patient medications, how can a pharmacist use a plain printout of the patient's pharmacy records?
8. For facilities such as long-term care (LTC), the pharmacy provides various printed records. How do the forms provided to an assisted living facility (ALF) differ for recording use of medications? (Visit *www.med-pass.com* and click on the **Assisted Living** button on the left side, then select the **Products** tab.)
9. Which records would be used most often in a skilled nursing facility (SNF)? Why are more forms used in the SNF than in retail?
10. Discuss the future of the printed records compared to electronic records.

APPENDIX A

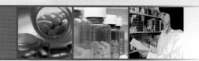

Sample Forms

There are many types of orders which a pharmacy technician may work with other than the regular prescription received at a doctor's office visit. The pharmacy technician in the community or retail pharmacy will routinely work with prescriptions brought in by the patient (customer), faxed, or emailed.

However, there are many more forms that are used to order medications. A few of the different forms are included in this appendix.

ADMINISTRATION RECORD

DATE
05/16/XX

Resident Name: ROUTINE, ORDERS

MAY05

ORDERS | FREQ. | 1 2 3 4 5 6 7 8 9 10 11 12 13 14 15 16 17 18 19 20 21 22 23 24 25 26 27 28 29 30 31

D/C   Order# 00016
01) (_) -PPD MANTOUX: TEST ID NOW AND IF NEGATIVE
REPEAT IN 7 DAYS AND ANNUALLY.
MONTH: _____ (S-CTPPD)

D/C   Order# 00017
02) (_) -PNEUMOVAX: INJECT 0.5ML IM OR SC X1 DOSE
IF NOT RECEIVED IN LAST 5 YEARS

D/C   Order# 00018
03) (_) -TETANUS TOXOID ADSORBED: INJECT 0.5ML IM
X1 DOSE IF NOT GIVEN IN LAST 10 YEARS

1 2 3 4 5 6 7 8 9 10 11 12 13 14 15 16 17 18 19 20 21 22 23 24 25 26 27 28 29 30 31

DIAGNOSIS

DOCTOR

RESIDENT

DATE

ROOM #

ALLERGIES

REVIEW OF ENTIRE DRUG REGIMEN
AND COMPREHENSIVE RESIDENT
CARE PLAN IS COMPLETED.

ANY IRREGULARITIES ARE DOCUMENTED
IN THE PHARMACIST'S MONTHLY REPORTS.

☐ NO IRREGULARITIES NOTED
☐ INSIGNIFICANT IRREGULARITIES NOTED
☐ SIGNIFICANT IRREGULARITIES NOTED

X _____
PHARMACY

_____ DATE

See Reverse Side For Verifying Signatures

PRN Orders
RESIDENT "CHEEKS" MEDS

04/01/20XX

	15	16	17	18	19	20	21	22	23	24	25	26	27	28	29	30	1	2	3	4	5	6	7	8	9	10	11	12	13	14	31

01/25/20XX RX 309628
ACETAMINOPHEN 325MG TABLET   325MG
 -I.E. TYLENOL 325MG   325MG
1 TABLET EVERY 4hrs AS NEEDED ELEV. TEMP
>101F

FREQUENCY: (columns 15 16 17 18 19 20 21 22 23 24 25 26 27 28 29 30 1 2 3 4 5 6 7 8 9 10 11 12 13 14 31)

SE: Anemia; Thrombocytopenia; Agranulocytosis; Hepatitis;

01/25/20XX RX 309629
BISACODYL 10MG SUPPOSITORY

1 RECTALLY PRN CONSTIPATION IF MOM NOT
EFFECTIVE AFTER 24HRS

FREQUENCY: (columns 15 16 17 18 19 20 21 22 23 24 25 26 27 28 29 30 1 2 3 4 5 6 7 8 9 10 11 12 13 14 31)

SE: Perianal Irritation; Nausea; Belching; Diarrhea; Cramps;

01/25/20XX RX 309630
MILK OF MAGNESIA - PHILLIPS

30CC BY MOUTH DAILY AS NEEDED IF NO B.M.
AFTER 2 DAYS

FREQUENCY: (columns 15 16 17 18 19 20 21 22 23 24 25 26 27 28 29 30 1 2 3 4 5 6 7 8 9 10 11 12 13 14 31)

SE: Increased Thirst; Gas; Diarrhea; Stomach Cramps;

FREQUENCY:

FREQUENCY:

FREQUENCY:

FREQUENCY:

PHYSICIAN: JONES, WILLIAM   423-888-6364   PARKINSON'S; HTN; HX DEPRESSION W/ANXIETY; DELUSIONAL DISORDER;
ALT. PHYS: DR. J. SMITH   423-877-6365   CHF; IRON DEFICIENCY ANEMIA; HYPOKALEMIA; CONSTIPATION; EDEMA;
                               DOB- 05/06/1933
                               ADM- 12-AB467   WOOL; MOHAIR
                               ACC- 017001
                               RM# 212A   SAMPLE FACILITY - STATION 1

Page 1

COMMENTS

Instructions:

A. WHEN PRNS ARE GIVEN, EXPLAIN IN NURSES NOTES.

B. SUGGEST REFUSED / WITHHELD MEDICATION EXPLAINED IN NURSES MEDICATION NOTES.

Date	Time	Initial	Comments

Date	Time	Initial	Comments

FULL SIGNATURE	INITIALS	TITLE	FULL SIGNATURE	INITIALS	TITLE

FULL SIGNATURE	INITIALS	TITLE	FULL SIGNATURE	INITIALS	TITLE

See Reverse Side For Verifying Signatures

Routine Orders
RESIDENT "CHEEKS" MEDS

04/01/20XX

Page 1

	FREQUENCY:	15	16	17	18	19	20	21	22	23	24	25	26	27	28	29	30	1	2	3	4	5	6	7	8	9	10	11	12	13	14	31

01/25/20XX RX 309632
ARTIFICIAL TEARS 15CC DROPS
INSTILL 2 DROPS IN BOTH EYES TWO TIMES A DAY
— 09:00
— 18:00

01/25/20XX RX 309633   325MG
FERROUS SULFATE 325MG TAB
1 TABLET BY MOUTH TWICE DAILY WITH FOOD
— 10:00
— 16:00
SE: Stomach Pain/cramps; Constipation; Nausea; Vomiting; Diar

01/25/20XX RX 309634   40MG   40MG
FUROSEMIDE 40MG TABLET
-I.E. LASIX 40MG TABLET
1 TABLET BY MOUTH TWICE DAILY
— 08:00
— 18:00
SE: Orthostatic Hypotension; Hyponatremia; Hypokalemia

01/25/20XX RX 309635   20MEQ
K-DUR 20MEQ TABLET SA
1 TABLET BY MOUTH TWICE DAILY
— 09:00
— 17:00
SE: Vomiting; Gas; Diarrhea; Stomach Pain; Discomfort; Hyperk

01/25/20XX RX 309636   75MG
PLAVIX 75MG TABLET
ONE TABLET BY MOUTH ONCE DAILY
— 07:30
SE: Purpura; Upper Respiratory Infection; Pain; Chest Pain

04/23/20XX
DO -NOT- RESUSCITATE

LOA WITH SUPERVISION & MEDS

PHYSICIAN: JONES, WILLIAM   423-888-6364   PARKINSON'S; HTN; HX DEPRESSION W/ANXIETY; DELUSIONAL DISORDER;
ALT. PHYS: DR. J. SMITH   423-877-6365   CHF; IRON DEFICIENCY ANEMIA; HYPOKALEMIA; CONSTIPATION; EDEMA;
                            DOB- 05/06/1933
                            ADM- 12-AB467   WOOL; MOHAIR
                            ACC- 017001
                            RM#   212A   SAMPLE FACILITY - STATION 1

Nurse's Medication Notes

Instructions:

A. SUGGEST REFUSED / WITHHELD MEDICATION
EXPLAINED IN NURSES MEDICATION NOTES.

B. WHEN PRN MEDICATIONS ARE GIVEN,
EXPLAIN IN NURSES MEDICATION NOTES.

Indicate Site With Appropriate Number:

1. BUTTOCKS (GLUTEUS) LEFT
2. BUTTOCKS (GLUTEUS) RIGHT
3. ARM (DELTOID) LEFT
4. ARM (DELTOID) RIGHT

5. THIGH (QUADRICEPS) LEFT
6. THIGH (QUADRICEPS) RIGHT
7. ABDOMEN LEFT
8. ABDOMEN RIGHT

9. UPPER BACK LEFT
10. UPPER BACK RIGHT
11. UPPER CHEST LEFT
12. UPPER CHEST RIGHT

RESULT CODES

B = BM RESULTED	N = SEE NURSES NOTES
E = EFFECTIVE	R = WITH RELIEF
I = INEFFECTIVE	S = SLEEP RESULTED

Date	Time	Init.	Drug - Strength - Dose	Site	Reason	Result	Date	Time	Obser. Init.

Initials	Signature & Title	Initials	Signature & Title

Date	Time	Init.	Drug - Strength - Dose	Site	Reason	Result	Date	Time	Obser. Init.

Initials	Signature & Title	Initials	Signature & Title

See Reverse Side For Verifying Signatures

04/01/20XX

Treatment Orders
RESIDENT "CHEEKS" MEDS

Page 1

01/25/20XX RX 310243
ARISTOCORT A 0.1% CREAM   0.1%

APPLY TO RASH ON FOREHEAD AS NEEDED -
ITCHING

FREQUENCY: 15 16 17 18 19 20 21 22 23 24 25 26 27 28 29 30 1 2 3 4 5 6 7 8 9 10 11 12 13 14 31
P
R
N

SE: Purpura; Telangiectasia; Furunculosis; Pyoderma; Skin Inf

01/25/20XX
APPLY VASELINE LOTION TO ELBOWS AND
KNEES TWICE DAILY

FREQUENCY: 15 16 17 18 19 20 21 22 23 24 25 26 27 28 29 30 1 2 3 4 5 6 7 8 9 10 11 12 13 14 31
7AM
3PM

01/27/20XX
APPLY TED HOSE (THIGH HIGH) EVERY MORNING
AND REMOVE AT BEDTIME

FREQUENCY: 15 16 17 18 19 20 21 22 23 24 25 26 27 28 29 30 1 2 3 4 5 6 7 8 9 10 11 12 13 14 31
ON
OFF

FREQUENCY:

FREQUENCY:

FREQUENCY:

FREQUENCY:

PHYSICIAN: JONES, WILLIAM   423-888-6364
ALT. PHYS: DR. J. SMITH   423-877-6365
                                   DOB- 05/06/1933
                                   ADM- 12-AB467
                                   ACC- 017001
                                   RM#   212A

PARKINSON'S; HTN; HX DEPRESSION W/ANXIETY; DELUSIONAL DISORDER;
CHF; IRON DEFICIENCY ANEMIA; HYPOKALEMIA; CONSTIPATION; EDEMA;

WOOL; MOHAIR

SAMPLE FACILITY - STATION 1

PHYSICIAN'S ORDER

Resident ROUTINE, ORDERS
Name:

DATE
05/16/XX   MAY05

ORDERS	FREQ.	OTHER ODERS

ACTIVITIES AND MOBILITY:
(_)-YES. (_)-NO.............. PHYSICAL
&.SOCIAL.ACTIVITIES.AS TOLERATED
(_)-WITH.ASSIST.OR.DEVICE (_)-BED.TO.CHAIR.
(_)-UP.IN.CHAIR-FREQUENCY_____ (S-CTACTIV)

D/C _____ Order# 00016
01) (_)-PPD MANTOUX: TEST ID NOW AND IF NEGATIVE
REPEAT IN 7 DAYS AND ANNUALLY.
MONTH:_____ (S-CTPPD)
ICD9
Diagnosis

(_)-YES.(_)-NO........... LEAVE OF ABSENCE AS
NEEDED (S-CTLOA)

D/C _____ Order# 00017
02) (_)-PNEUMOVAX: INJECT 0.5ML IM OR SC X1 DOSE
IF NOT RECEIVED IN LAST 5 YEARS
ICD9
Diagnosis

CONSULTATIONS & THERAPIES:
PODIATRY, DENTAL, OPHTHALMIC.. CONSULTATIONS
AS.NEEDED OTHER: _____
(S-CTCONSULT)

D/C _____ Order# 00018
03) (_)-TETANUS TOXOID ADSORBED: INJECT 0.5ML IM
X1 DOSE IF NOT GIVEN IN LAST 10 YEARS
ICD9
Diagnosis

UNIVERSAL ORDERS:
DR ORDERS, PATIENT CARE PLAN, ACTIVITIES &
DISCHARGE REVIEWED & APPROVED

NURSE MAY CHECK FOR CONSTIPATION AND PROVIDE
DIGITAL STIMULATION AS NEEDED

ICD9
Diagnosis

MAY CHANGE BETWEEN ORAL SOLIDS / LIQUIDS / OPEN
CAPSULES OR CRUSH TABS UNLESS CONTRAINDICATED
OR GIVE VIA ENTERAL TUBE IF TUBE IN PLACE

ICD9
Diagnosis

DIETARY CONSISTENCY MAY BE CHANGED AS CONDITION
WARRANTS

MAY BATHE IN CENTURY TUB, SHOWER OR WHIRLPOOL

ICD9
Diagnosis

WEIGHT: RECORD AT LEAST EACH MONTH & REPORT 5%
DIFFERENCE TO PHYSICIAN

URINARY CATHETER ORDERS:
MAY STRAIGHT CATH TO OBTAIN U/A AS NEEDED
(S-CTCATH)

ICD9
Diagnosis

ROUTINE ORDERS:

.

.

ICD9
Diagnosis

.

DIAGNOSIS

.

.

DOCTOR   DATE
                    ROOM #
RESIDENT   ALLERGIES

PRESCRIBER SIGNATURE _____   DATE _____

REVIEWED BY _____ DATE _____   NOTED BY _____   DATE _____

TOTAL RX: 0	TOTAL ROUTINES: 0	TOTAL PRN: 0	REVIEW OF ENTIRE DRUG REGIMEN AND COMPREHENSIVE RESIDENT CARE PLAN IS COMPLETED.	☐ NO IRREGULARITIES NOTED
	TOTAL RTN TRMT: 0	TOTAL PRN TRMT: 0		☐ INSIGNIFICANT IRREGULARITIES NOTED
*			ANY IRREGULARITIES ARE DOCUMENTED IN THE PHARMACIST'S MONTHLY REPORTS.	☐ SIGNIFICANT IRREGULARITIES NOTED
*			X	
			PHARMACY	DATE

☐ SEND * MEDS ONLY   ☐ SEND NO MEDS   ☐ SEND ALL MEDS

FIN PLAN-   SEX- M   DOB-
  NH RES#-   RES CODE- 96027

ROUTINE, ORDERS

Medication Administration Record (MAR)

MO/YR: _____   Facility Name: _____

Medication	Start/Stop Date	Hour	1	2	3	4	5	6	7	8	9	10	11	12	13	14	15	16	17	18	19	20	21	22	23	24	25	26	27	28	29	30	31
	Start																																	
	Stop																																	
	Start																																	
	Stop																																	
	Start																																	
	Stop																																	
	Start																																	
	Stop																																	
	Start																																	
	Stop																																	
	Start																																	
	Stop																																	

Diagnosis: _____

DIET (Special Instructions, e.g. Texture, Bite Size, Position, etc.) _____

Allergies: _____

Physician Name _____

Phone Number _____

Comments

A. Put initials in appropriate box when medication is given.
B. Circle initials when not given.
C. State reason for refusal / omission on back of form.
D. PRN Medications: Reason given and results must be noted on back of form.
E. Legend: S = School; H = Home visit; W = Work; P = Program.

Record # _____

NAME: _____   Date of Birth: _____   Sex: _____

VITAL SIGNS	1	2	3	4	5	6	7	8	9	10	11	12	13	14	15	16	17	18	19	20	21	22	23	24	25	26	27	28	29	30	31
TEMPERATURE																															
PULSE																															
RESPIRATION																															
WEIGHT																															

PRN AND MEDICATIONS NOT ADMINSTERED

Date	Hour	Initials	Medication	Reason	Result		Initials	Staff Signature
						1		
						2		
						3		
						4		
						5		
						6		
						7		
						8		
						9		
						10		
						11		
						12		
						13		
						14		
						15		
						16		
						17		
						18		
						19		

Name

MO/ YR

MEDICATION RECONCILIATION ORDER FORM

PATIENT NAME:

UNIT NUMBER:

Allergies:

LIST BELOW ALL OF THE PATIENT'S MEDICATIONS <u>PRIOR TO ADMISSION</u> INCLUDING OTC AND ALTERNATIVE MEDS
(ALTERNATIVE MEDICATIONS WILL NOT BE CONTINUED ON ADMISSION)
NEW MEDICATIONS OR MEDICATION CHANGES SHOULD BE WRITTEN ON ADMISSION ORDERS

PROHIBITED ABBREVIATIONS: qd, qod, U, IU, .X, X.0, MS, MSO4, MgSO4, µg, OD, OS, OU, AD, AS, AU, tiw

Source of Medication list: (check all used)

☐ Patient medication list
☐ Patient/Family recall
☐ Pharmacy _____
☐ Primary care physician list / PCHIS
☐ Previous discharge paperwork
☐ Medication Administration Record from facility
☐ Other:

☐ **CHECK HERE IF THIS IS AN ADDENDUM TO OR REVISION OF PREVIOUSLY COMPLETED MEDICATION LIST**

☐ Pregnant?
☐ Breastfeeding?

CIRCLE C to continue
OR
DC to discontinue

MEDICATION HISTORY RECORDED/VERIFIED WITH PATIENT BY: _____

DATE RECORDED: _____

MEDICATION NAME (WRITE LEGIBLY)	DOSE (mg, mcg)	ROUTE (PO, GT, SC, IV)	FREQUENCY	LAST DOSE DATE/TIME	PHYSICIAN ORDER — CONTINUE ON ADMISSION	
1.					C	DC
2.					C	DC
3.					C	DC
4.					C	DC
5.					C	DC
6.					C	DC
7.					C	DC
8.					C	DC
9.					C	DC
10.					C	DC
11.					C	DC
12.					C	DC
13.					C	DC

Do not scan or take off orders without MD/NP/PA signature

Signature MD/DO/NP/PA_____Printed Name_____Pager #_____Date_____

Signature RN_____Printed Name_____Date_____

Reviewed on Transfer: ☐   By: _____   Date: _____
Reviewed on Discharge: ☐   By: _____   Date: _____

Scan to Pharmacy. File under Orders.

Instructions for proper use:

Admission:

1. A nurse, mid-level provider, or physician should take as thorough a medication history as possible. Consultation with the primary care physician, pharmacy, and family members may be necessary to generate the most accurate medication list.

2. **Upon admission**, the physician/nurse practitioner/physician's assistant responsible for the patient should carefully consider whether to continue (C) or Discontinue (DC) each medication and circle the appropriate letters..

   a. For medications that require dosage changes, the medication should be discontinued on this form, and the new dosage should be written on the admission order sheet.

   b. For medications for which there exists a hospital therapeutic substitution, the medication should be discontinued and the new medication to be substituted should be ordered on the admission order form.

3. Upon completion, the provider should sign and date on the M.D. signature line. This is now treated as a physician's order. The form is scanned to pharmacy and filed in the Orders section of the chart.

4. The nurse confirms the history with the patient and confirms proper transcription to the written Medication Administration record (Kardex) and signs on the Nurse signature line.

5. Admission orders should indicate, "See medication reconciliation form." All new medications to be started on admission should appear on the admission order form. The History and Physical may indicate "See reconciliation form" in the Medications area.

6. If additional medication history is made available after the form has already been scanned to pharmacy, the medication history may be updated by completing a second reconciliation form noting the addition or changes, and checking the Addendum/Revision box.

Transfer:

7. Upon transfer, this form should be reviewed together with the Medication Administration Record (Kardex). The provider should carefully consider whether each medication should be continued, resumed, or discontinued after the patient moves to another area within the hospital. All medications need to be reordered.

Discharge:

8. At discharge, this form should be reviewed together with the Medication Administration Record (Kardex). The provider should carefully consider whether each medication should be continued, resumed, or discontinued after the patient leaves the hospital. All medications and instructions should also be recorded on the discharge paperwork.

Prohibited Abbreviation	Potential Problem	Preferred Term
U (for unit)	Mistaken as zero, four or cc.	Write "**unit**"
IU (for international unit)	Mistaken as IV (intravenous) or 10 (ten).	Write "**international unit**" or "**unit**"
Q.D., Q.O.D. (any form)	Mistaken for each other. The period after the Q can be mistaken for an "I" and the O can be mistaken for an "I".	Write "**daily**" and "**every other day**"
Trailing zero (**X.0 mg**), Lack of leading zero (**.X mg**)	Decimal point is missed.	Never write a zero by itself after a decimal point (**X mg**), and always use a zero before a decimal point (**0.X mg**)
MS, MSO$_4$, MgSO4	Confused for one another.	Write "**morphine sulfate**" or "**magnesium sulfate**"
µg (for microgram)	Mistaken for mg (milligrams) resulting in one thousandfold dosing overdose.	Write "**mcg**"
T.I.W. (for three times a week)	Mistaken for three times a day or twice weekly resulting in an overdose.	Write "**3 times weekly**" or "**three times weekly**"
A.S., A.D., A.U. O.S., O.D., O.U.	Mistaken for each other	Write: "**left ear**," "**right ear**" or "**both ears**;" "**left eye**," "**right eye**," or "**both eyes**"

HT: _____ cm **WT:** _____ kg

Adult *Total* Parenteral Nutrition Order Form *(Central Line Only)*

Date Time	Is *central* line access in place? ☐ No ☐ Yes Type _____ Date placed _____

Please note: Prescribers must make selections in sections 1-6 of form

1. Base Formula(Check one)	2. Infusion Schedule
☐ Standard Base: dextrose 20% and amino acids (AA) 4.25% 　　(D40W 500 mL and AA 8.5% 500 mL) ☐ Individualized base: Dextrose _____% and AA _____%: 　　(final concentration) 　　　　**OR** 　　Dextrose _____% _____ mL 　　AA　　_____% _____ mL 　　_____	Rate: _____mL/hour _____ **Cycling Schedule (home TPN only)** Cycle _____mL fluid over _____hours Begin at _____

3. Standard Electrolytes/Additives	OR Specify Individualized Electrolytes/ Additives	
Check here ☐	**Specify amount of electrolyte.**	**Check all that apply**
NaCl　　　40 mEq / L	NaCl _____ mEq / L	☐ Adult MVI 10 mLs / day
NaAc　　　20 mEq / L	NaAc _____ mEq / L	☐ MTE – 5 　3 mLs / day
KCl　　　　20 mEq / L	NaPhos _____ mEq / L	☐ Regular Human Insulin _____units / Liter
Kphos　　 22 mEq / L	KCl _____ mEq / L	☐ Vitamin C 500 mg / day
CaGlu　　 4.7 mEq / L	KAc _____ mEq / L	☐ H 2 antagonist _____mg / day drug _____
MagSO4　 8 mEq / L	Kphos _____ mEq / L	☐ Other additives
Adult MVI　10 mLs / day	CaGlu _____ mEq / L	
MTE-5　　 3 mLs/ day	Mag SO4 _____ mEq / L	
DO NOT USE IN RENAL DYSFUNCTION!	**Maximum Phosphate (Na phos 40 mEq / L or K phos 44 mEq / L) and maximum calcium 10 mEq / L**	_____ _____ _____

4. Lipids (Check one)	5. Blood Glucose monitoring orders
Infuse lipids over 12 hours IV ☐ 20% 250 mL every Tuesday/Thursday ☐ 20% 250 mL every day ☐ 20% 250 mL every other day ☐ Other schedule _____ _____	Blood glucose monitoring every_____ hour(s) with sliding scale regular human insulin. Route (Circle one) **SQ**　　**IV** **Sliding scale** (Check one) ☐ Sliding scale per P and T protocol ☐ Individualized sliding scale (write below) _____ _____ _____ _____

Additional Orders (All patients)	6. Routine Laboratory Orders (Check all that apply)
1. Consult Nutrition Support Team. 2. CMP, Mg, Phos, triglyceride, prealbumin in the AM 3. Weigh patient daily. 4. Strict I/O & document in chart. 5. Keep TPN line inviolate. 6. If TPN interrupted for any reason, hang D10W@ current TPN rate.	☐ BMP, Mg, Phos every AM X 3 days then every Monday & Thursday. ☐ Prealbumin every Monday ☐ Metabolic study per RT (University only) ☐ 24 hour UUN and creatinine clearance

Physician Signature

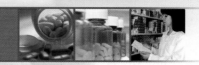

Health Insurance Claim Form (CMS-1500) Completion Instructions

Health Insurance Claim Form (CMS-1500) Completion Instructions

Claims must be submitted on the CMS-1500 for professional services. The following information is **required** on every claim:

BOX 1	Indicate that this is a TRICARE claim by checking the box under "TRICARE CHAMPUS."
BOX 1a	Sponsor's Social Security number. The sponsor is the person that qualifies the patient for TRICARE benefits.
BOX 2	Patient's name
BOX 3	Patient's date of birth and sex
BOX 4	Sponsor's full name. Do not complete if "self" is checked in BOX 6.
BOX 5	Patient's address including ZIP code. This must be a physical address. Post office boxes are not acceptable.
BOX 6	Patient's relationship to sponsor
BOX 7	Sponsor's address including ZIP code
BOX 8	Marital and employment status of patient

Note: Box 11d should be completed prior to determining the need for completing Boxes 9a through 9d. If Box 11d is checked "yes," Boxes 9a and 9d must be completed. In addition, if there is another insurance carrier, the mailing address of that insurance carrier must be attached to the claim form.

BOX 9	Full name of person with other health insurance (OHI) that covers patient
BOX 9a	Other insured's policy or group number
BOX 9b	Other insured's date of birth and sex (*Not required, but preferred*)
BOX 9c	Other insured's employer name or name of school
BOX 9d	Name of insurance plan or program name where individual has OHI
BOX 10a-c	Check to indicate whether employment or accident related. (*In the case of an auto accident, indicate the state where it occurred.*)

Note: Box 11 through Box 11c questions pertain to the sponsor.

BOX 11	Indicate policy group or Federal Employees Compensation Act (FECA) number (*if applicable*).
BOX 11a	Sponsor's date of birth and sex, if different than Box 3
BOX 11b	Sponsor's branch of service
BOX 11c	Indicate "TRICARE" in this field.
BOX 11d	Indicate if there is another health insurance plan primary to TRICARE in this field.
BOX 12	Patient's or authorized person's signature and date; release of information. A signature on the file is acceptable provided signature is updated annually.
BOX 13	Insured's or Authorized Person's Signature. This authorizes payment to the physician or supplier.
BOX 14	Date of current illness or injury/ Date of pregnancy (*Required for injury or pregnancy*)
BOX 15	First date (*MM/DD/YY*) had same or similar illness (*Not required, but preferred*)
BOX 16	Dates patient unable to work (*Not required, but preferred*)
BOX 17	Name of referring physician (*Very important to include this information*)
BOX 17a	Identification (*non-NPI*) number of referring physician with qualifier
BOX 17b	Referring physician NPI
BOX 18	Admit and discharge date of hospitalization
BOX 19	Referral number
BOX 20	Check if lab work was performed outside the physician's office and indicate charges by the lab. If an outside provider (*e.g., laboratory*) performs a service, claims should include modifier "90" or indicate "Yes" in this block.
BOX 21	Indicate at least one, and up to four, specific diagnosis codes.
BOX 23	Prior authorization number
BOX 24A	Date of service
BOX 24B	Place of service
BOX 24C	EMG (emergency) indicator

BOX 24D	CPT/HCPC procedure code with modifier, if applicable
BOX 24E	Diagnosis code reference number (*pointer*)
BOX 24F	Charges for listed service
BOX 24G	Days or units for each line item
BOX 24H	Early and Periodic Screening, Diagnosis, and Treatment (EPSDT) related services/Family planning response and appropriate reason code (*if applicable*)
BOX 24I	Qualifier identifying if the number is a non-NPI ID
BOX 24J	Rendering Provider ID number. Enter the non-NPI ID number in the shaded area. Enter the NPI number in the unshaded area.
BOX 25	Physician's/Supplier's Tax Identification Number
BOX 26	Patient's Account Number (*Not required, but preferred*)
BOX 27	Indicate whether provider accepts TRICARE assignment.
BOX 28	Total charges submitted on claim
BOX 29	Amount paid by patient or other carrier
BOX 30	Amount due after other payments are applied (*Required if OHI*)
BOX 31	Authorized signature
BOX 32	Name and address where services were rendered. This **must** be the actual physical location. If you use an independent billing service, please **do not** use this address.
BOX 32a	NPI of the service facility location
BOX 32b	Two-digit qualifier identifying the non-NPI number followed by the ID number (*if necessary*)
BOX 33	Physician's/Supplier's billing name, address, ZIP code, and phone number
BOX 33a	NPI of billing provider
BOX 33b	Two-digit qualifier identifying the non-NPI number followed by the ID number (*if necessary*)

CMS-1500 Place of Service Codes

11	Office
12	Home
15	Mobile unit
21	Inpatient hospital
22	Outpatient hospital
23	Emergency room—hospital
24	Ambulatory surgical center
25	Birthing center
26	Military treatment facility (MTF)
31	Skilled nursing facility
32	Nursing facility
33	Custodial care facility
34	Hospice
41	Ambulance, land
42	Ambulance, air or water
51	Inpatient psychiatric facility
52	Psychiatric facility, partial hospitalization
53	Community mental health center
54	Intermediate care center/mentally retarded
55	Residential substance abuse treatment facility
56	Psychiatric residential treatment center
61	Comprehensive inpatient rehabilitation facility
62	Comprehensive outpatient rehabilitation facility
65	End-stage renal disease treatment facility
71	State or local public health clinic
72	Rural health clinic
81	Independent laboratory
99	Other unlisted facility

Type of Service Codes

1	Medical care
2	Surgery
3	Consultation
4	Diagnostic X-ray
5	Diagnostic laboratory
6	Radiation therapy
7	Anesthesia
8	Assistant at surgery
9	Other medical service
A	Durable medical equipment (DME) rental/purchase
B	Drugs
C	Ambulatory surgery
D	Hospice
E	Second opinion on elective surgery
F	Maternity
G	Dental
H	Mental health care
I	Ambulance
J	Extended Care Health Option (ECHO)/Program for Persons with Disabilities (PFPWD)

1500

HEALTH INSURANCE CLAIM FORM

APPROVED BY NATIONAL UNIFORM CLAIM COMMITTEE 08/05

CARRIER →

☐☐ PICA

PICA ☐☐

1. ☐ MEDICARE (Medicare #) ☐ MEDICAID (Medicaid #) ☐ TRICARE CHAMPUS (Sponsor's SSN) ☐ CHAMPVA (Member ID#) ☐ GROUP HEALTH PLAN (SSN or ID) ☐ FECA BLK LUNG (SSN) ☐ OTHER (ID)

1a. INSURED'S I.D. NUMBER   (For Program in Item 1)

2. PATIENT'S NAME (Last Name, First Name, Middle Initial)

3. PATIENT'S BIRTH DATE MM | DD | YY   SEX M ☐ F ☐

4. INSURED'S NAME (Last Name, First Name, Middle Initial)

5. PATIENT'S ADDRESS (No., Street)

6. PATIENT RELATIONSHIP TO INSURED Self ☐ Spouse ☐ Child ☐ Other ☐

7. INSURED'S ADDRESS (No., Street)

CITY   STATE

8. PATIENT STATUS Single ☐ Married ☐ Other ☐

Employed ☐ Full-Time Student ☐ Part-Time Student ☐

CITY   STATE

ZIP CODE   TELEPHONE (Include Area Code) (   )

ZIP CODE   TELEPHONE (Include Area Code) (   )

9. OTHER INSURED'S NAME (Last Name, First Name, Middle Initial)

10. IS PATIENT'S CONDITION RELATED TO:

11. INSURED'S POLICY GROUP OR FECA NUMBER

a. OTHER INSURED'S POLICY OR GROUP NUMBER

a. EMPLOYMENT? (Current or Previous) ☐ YES ☐ NO

a. INSURED'S DATE OF BIRTH MM | DD | YY   SEX M ☐ F ☐

b. OTHER INSURED'S DATE OF BIRTH MM | DD | YY   SEX M ☐ F ☐

b. AUTO ACCIDENT? PLACE (State) ☐ YES ☐ NO

b. EMPLOYER'S NAME OR SCHOOL NAME

c. EMPLOYER'S NAME OR SCHOOL NAME

c. OTHER ACCIDENT? ☐ YES ☐ NO

c. INSURANCE PLAN NAME OR PROGRAM NAME

d. INSURANCE PLAN NAME OR PROGRAM NAME

10d. RESERVED FOR LOCAL USE

d. IS THERE ANOTHER HEALTH BENEFIT PLAN? ☐ YES ☐ NO   If yes, return to and complete item 9 a-d.

READ BACK OF FORM BEFORE COMPLETING & SIGNING THIS FORM.

12. PATIENT'S OR AUTHORIZED PERSON'S SIGNATURE I authorize the release of any medical or other information necessary to process this claim. I also request payment of government benefits either to myself or to the party who accepts assignment below.

SIGNED _____ DATE _____

13. INSURED'S OR AUTHORIZED PERSON'S SIGNATURE I authorize payment of medical benefits to the undersigned physician or supplier for services described below.

SIGNED _____

14. DATE OF CURRENT: MM | DD | YY ILLNESS (First symptom) OR INJURY (Accident) OR PREGNANCY(LMP)

15. IF PATIENT HAS HAD SAME OR SIMILAR ILLNESS. GIVE FIRST DATE MM | DD | YY

16. DATES PATIENT UNABLE TO WORK IN CURRENT OCCUPATION MM | DD | YY FROM   TO MM | DD | YY

17. NAME OF REFERRING PROVIDER OR OTHER SOURCE

17a.
17b. NPI

18. HOSPITALIZATION DATES RELATED TO CURRENT SERVICES MM | DD | YY FROM   TO MM | DD | YY

19. RESERVED FOR LOCAL USE

20. OUTSIDE LAB? ☐ YES ☐ NO $ CHARGES

21. DIAGNOSIS OR NATURE OF ILLNESS OR INJURY (Relate Items 1, 2, 3 or 4 to Item 24E by Line)

1. L___ . ___   3. L___ . ___
2. L___ . ___   4. L___ . ___

22. MEDICAID RESUBMISSION CODE   ORIGINAL REF. NO.

23. PRIOR AUTHORIZATION NUMBER

24. A. DATE(S) OF SERVICE From MM DD YY To MM DD YY | B. PLACE OF SERVICE | C. EMG | D. PROCEDURES, SERVICES, OR SUPPLIES (Explain Unusual Circumstances) CPT/HCPCS MODIFIER | E. DIAGNOSIS POINTER | F. $ CHARGES | G. DAYS OR UNITS | H. EPSDT Family Plan | I. ID. QUAL. | J. RENDERING PROVIDER ID. #

1 | | | | | | | | | | NPI

2 | | | | | | | | | | NPI

3 | | | | | | | | | | NPI

4 | | | | | | | | | | NPI

5 | | | | | | | | | | NPI

6 | | | | | | | | | | NPI

25. FEDERAL TAX I.D. NUMBER ☐ SSN ☐ EIN

26. PATIENT'S ACCOUNT NO.

27. ACCEPT ASSIGNMENT? (For govt. claims, see back) ☐ YES ☐ NO

28. TOTAL CHARGE $

29. AMOUNT PAID $

30. BALANCE DUE $

31. SIGNATURE OF PHYSICIAN OR SUPPLIER INCLUDING DEGREES OR CREDENTIALS (I certify that the statements on the reverse apply to this bill and are made a part thereof.)

SIGNED _____ DATE _____

32. SERVICE FACILITY LOCATION INFORMATION

a. NPI   b.

33. BILLING PROVIDER INFO & PH # (   )

a. NPI   b.

PATIENT AND INSURED INFORMATION

PHYSICIAN OR SUPPLIER INFORMATION

NUCC Instruction Manual available at: www.nucc.org   **PLEASE PRINT OR TYPE**   APPROVED OMB-0938-0999 FORM CMS-1500 (08-05)

BECAUSE THIS FORM IS USED BY VARIOUS GOVERNMENT AND PRIVATE HEALTH PROGRAMS, SEE SEPARATE INSTRUCTIONS ISSUED BY APPLICABLE PROGRAMS.

NOTICE: Any person who knowingly files a statement of claim containing any misrepresentation or any false, incomplete or misleading information may be guilty of a criminal act punishable under law and may be subject to civil penalties.

REFERS TO GOVERNMENT PROGRAMS ONLY

MEDICARE AND CHAMPUS PAYMENTS: A patient's signature requests that payment be made and authorizes release of any information necessary to process the claim and certifies that the information provided in Blocks 1 through 12 is true, accurate and complete. In the case of a Medicare claim, the patient's signature authorizes any entity to release to Medicare medical and nonmedical information, including employment status, and whether the person has employer group health insurance, liability, no-fault, worker's compensation or other insurance which is responsible to pay for the services for which the Medicare claim is made. See 42 CFR 411.24(a). If item 9 is completed, the patient's signature authorizes release of the information to the health plan or agency shown. In Medicare assigned or CHAMPUS participation cases, the physician agrees to accept the charge determination of the Medicare carrier or CHAMPUS fiscal intermediary as the full charge, and the patient is responsible only for the deductible, coinsurance and noncovered services. Coinsurance and the deductible are based upon the charge determination of the Medicare carrier or CHAMPUS fiscal intermediary if this is less than the charge submitted. CHAMPUS is not a health insurance program but makes payment for health benefits provided through certain affiliations with the Uniformed Services. Information on the patient's sponsor should be provided in those items captioned in "Insured"; i.e., items 1a, 4, 6, 7, 9, and 11.

BLACK LUNG AND FECA CLAIMS

The provider agrees to accept the amount paid by the Government as payment in full. See Black Lung and FECA instructions regarding required procedure and diagnosis coding systems.

SIGNATURE OF PHYSICIAN OR SUPPLIER (MEDICARE, CHAMPUS, FECA AND BLACK LUNG)

I certify that the services shown on this form were medically indicated and necessary for the health of the patient and were personally furnished by me or were furnished incident to my professional service by my employee under my immediate personal supervision, except as otherwise expressly permitted by Medicare or CHAMPUS regulations.

For services to be considered as "incident" to a physician's professional service, 1) they must be rendered under the physician's immediate personal supervision by his/her employee, 2) they must be an integral, although incidental part of a covered physician's service, 3) they must be of kinds commonly furnished in physician's offices, and 4) the services of nonphysicians must be included on the physician's bills.

For CHAMPUS claims, I further certify that I (or any employee) who rendered services am not an active duty member of the Uniformed Services or a civilian employee of the United States Government or a contract employee of the United States Government, either civilian or military (refer to 5 USC 5536). For Black-Lung claims, I further certify that the services performed were for a Black Lung-related disorder.

No Part B Medicare benefits may be paid unless this form is received as required by existing law and regulations (42 CFR 424.32).

NOTICE: Any one who misrepresents or falsifies essential information to receive payment from Federal funds requested by this form may upon conviction be subject to fine and imprisonment under applicable Federal laws.

NOTICE TO PATIENT ABOUT THE COLLECTION AND USE OF MEDICARE, CHAMPUS, FECA, AND BLACK LUNG INFORMATION
(PRIVACY ACT STATEMENT)

We are authorized by CMS, CHAMPUS and OWCP to ask you for information needed in the administration of the Medicare, CHAMPUS, FECA, and Black Lung programs. Authority to collect information is in section 205(a), 1862, 1872 and 1874 of the Social Security Act as amended, 42 CFR 411.24(a) and 424.5(a) (6), and 44 USC 3101;41 CFR 101 et seq and 10 USC 1079 and 1086; 5 USC 8101 et seq; and 30 USC 901 et seq; 38 USC 613; E.O. 9397.

The information we obtain to complete claims under these programs is used to identify you and to determine your eligibility. It is also used to decide if the services and supplies you received are covered by these programs and to insure that proper payment is made.

The information may also be given to other providers of services, carriers, intermediaries, medical review boards, health plans, and other organizations or Federal agencies, for the effective administration of Federal provisions that require other third parties payers to pay primary to Federal program, and as otherwise necessary to administer these programs. For example, it may be necessary to disclose information about the benefits you have used to a hospital or doctor. Additional disclosures are made through routine uses for information contained in systems of records.

FOR MEDICARE CLAIMS: See the notice modifying system No. 09-70-0501, titled, 'Carrier Medicare Claims Record,' published in the Federal Register, Vol. 55 No. 177, page 37549, Wed. Sept. 12, 1990, or as updated and republished.

FOR OWCP CLAIMS: Department of Labor, Privacy Act of 1974, "Republication of Notice of Systems of Records," Federal Register Vol. 55 No. 40, Wed Feb. 28, 1990, See ESA-5, ESA-6, ESA-12, ESA-13, ESA-30, or as updated and republished.

FOR CHAMPUS CLAIMS: PRINCIPLE PURPOSE(S): To evaluate eligibility for medical care provided by civilian sources and to issue payment upon establishment of eligibility and determination that the services/supplies received are authorized by law.

ROUTINE USE(S): Information from claims and related documents may be given to the Dept. of Veterans Affairs, the Dept. of Health and Human Services and/or the Dept. of Transportation consistent with their statutory administrative responsibilities under CHAMPUS/CHAMPVA; to the Dept. of Justice for representation of the Secretary of Defense in civil actions; to the Internal Revenue Service, private collection agencies, and consumer reporting agencies in connection with recoupment claims; and to Congressional Offices in response to inquiries made at the request of the person to whom a record pertains. Appropriate disclosures may be made to other federal, state, local, foreign government agencies, private business entities, and individual providers of care, on matters relating to entitlement, claims adjudication, fraud, program abuse, utilization review, quality assurance, peer review, program integrity, third-party liability, coordination of benefits, and civil and criminal litigation related to the operation of CHAMPUS.

DISCLOSURES: Voluntary; however, failure to provide information will result in delay in payment or may result in denial of claim. With the one exception discussed below, there are no penalties under these programs for refusing to supply information. However, failure to furnish information regarding the medical services rendered or the amount charged would prevent payment of claims under these programs. Failure to furnish any other information, such as name or claim number, would delay payment of the claim. Failure to provide medical information under FECA could be deemed an obstruction.

It is mandatory that you tell us if you know that another party is responsible for paying for your treatment. Section 1128B of the Social Security Act and 31 USC 3801-3812 provide penalties for withholding this information.

You should be aware that P.L. 100-503, the "Computer Matching and Privacy Protection Act of 1988", permits the government to verify information by way of computer matches.

MEDICAID PAYMENTS (PROVIDER CERTIFICATION)

I hereby agree to keep such records as are necessary to disclose fully the extent of services provided to individuals under the State's Title XIX plan and to furnish information regarding any payments claimed for providing such services as the State Agency or Dept. of Health and Human Services may request.

I further agree to accept, as payment in full, the amount paid by the Medicaid program for those claims submitted for payment under that program, with the exception of authorized deductible, coinsurance, co-payment or similar cost-sharing charge.

SIGNATURE OF PHYSICIAN (OR SUPPLIER): I certify that the services listed above were medically indicated and necessary to the health of this patient and were personally furnished by me or my employee under my personal direction.

NOTICE: This is to certify that the foregoing information is true, accurate and complete. I understand that payment and satisfaction of this claim will be from Federal and State funds, and that any false claims, statements, or documents, or concealment of a material fact, may be prosecuted under applicable Federal or State laws.

According to the Paperwork Reduction Act of 1995, no persons are required to respond to a collection of information unless it displays a valid OMB control number. The valid OMB control number for this information collection is 0938-0999. The time required to complete this information collection is estimated to average 10 minutes per response, including the time to review instructions, search existing data resources, gather the data needed, and complete and review the information collection. If you have any comments concerning the accuracy of the time estimate(s) or suggestions for improving this form, please write to: CMS, Attn: PRA Reports Clearance Officer, 7500 Security Boulevard, Baltimore, Maryland 21244-1850. This address is for comments and/or suggestions only. DO NOT MAIL COMPLETED CLAIM FORMS TO THIS ADDRESS.

Sample of Pharmacy Provider Application

CBCA Rx PARTICIPATING PHARMACY PROVIDER APPLICATION

This document must be completed for all store locations of your Pharmacy.

General

Company Name

Street Address

Federal Tax ID #	State Pharmacy Operating License #
Pharmacy System	System Distributors License

Pharmacy Name

City	State	Zip
NABP #	Fax #	Telephone

Contact Person at Pharmacy

Services

1. What are your pharmacy hours of operation?

Monday	Tuesday	Wednesday	Thursday	Friday	Saturday	Sunday

2. Does your pharmacy offer a delivery service? ☐ Yes ☐ No

3. Does your pharmacy offer 24-hour emergency service? ☐ Yes ☐ No

4. Does your pharmacy provide compounding? ☐ Yes ☐ No

5. Do your employees have multilingual patient information needs? ☐ Yes ☐ No

6. Does your pharmacy system support multilingual patient information needs? ☐ Yes ☐ No

7. What other special service does your pharmacy offer? ☐ Yes ☐ No

License and Related Information

1. Does your pharmacy have a valid DEA registration Number? ☐ Yes ☐ No

2. Has your DEA number ever been suspended or revoked? ☐ Yes ☐ No

3. Has the Pharmacy, any pharmacist employed or its officers ever been convicted of a felony? ☐ Yes ☐ No

4. Has any individual provider been suspended or terminated from any Medicare or Medicaid programs in any state? ☐ Yes ☐ No

5. Does any individual provider have any impairment due to chemical dependency/drug abuse? ☐ Yes ☐ No

6. Does any individual provider have past or pending professional disciplinary actions, sanctions, or licensure limitations in the state in which the pharmacy operates? ☐ Yes ☐ No

7. Has an out-of-court settlement or a judgment been paid concerning a professional liability claim on behalf of your pharmacy by any malpractice carrier? ☐ Yes ☐ No

8. Please provide the following:
   - A copy of the Pharmacy's valid State Pharmacy Operating License;
   - Proof of valid professional liability and general liability insurance in the amounts of $1 million per occurence and $2 million aggregate coverage;
   - A copy of a valid DEA registration;
   - A copy of each Pharmacy's NABP number;
   - A completed Participating Pharmacy Provider Application;
   - A copy of any pharmacist license which has restrictions;
   - A copy of the patient information leaflet you provide Members with each prscription.

Pleas explain "yes" answers to any of questions 2 – 7 on attached sheet.

Labeling

Place a sample label used when filling prescriptions here:

Sample of Insurance Card

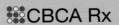

CBCA Rx   1-800-383-8737

Your Company, Inc.
Group #: xxxxx

Member Name: SUE FALLS
Member ID Number: 123456789

BIN# 006160

CBCA Rx
1-800-383-8737

Members:
You must present this card to a participating pharmacy when purchasing prescriptions.

For drug claim information or to locate the nearest participating pharmacy in your area, call 1-800-383-8737.

Pharmaciate:
For claims and eligibility questions call 1-800-383-8737.

NCPDP UNIVERSAL CLAIM FORM (UCF)

I.D.

GROUP I.D.

NAME

PLAN NAME

PATIENT NAME

OTHER COVERAGE CODE (1)

PERSON CODE (2)

PATIENT DATE OF BIRTH | PATIENT GENDER CODE (3)

MM   DD   CCYY

PATIENT RELATIONSHIP CODE (4)

PHARMACY NAME

ADDRESS

SERVICE PROVIDER I.D.   QUAL (5)

FOR OFFICE USE ONLY

CITY

PHONE NO.

(   )

STATE | ZIP CODE

FAX NO.

(   )

WORKERS COMP. INFORMATION

EMPLOYER NAME

ADDRESS

CITY

STATE

ZIP CODE

CARRIER I.D. (6) | EMPLOYER PHONE NO. | DATE OF INJURY | CLAIM REFERENCE I.D. (7)

(   )

MM   DD   CCYY

I have hereby read the Certification Statement on the reverse side. I hereby certify to and accept the terms thereof. I also certify that I have received 1 or 2 (please circle number) prescription(s) listed below.

PATIENT/AUTHORIZED REPRESENTATIVE

ATTENTION RECEIPT PLEASE READ CERTIFICATION STATEMENT ON REVERSE SIDE

1

PRESCRIPTION / SERV. REF. #	QUAL. (8)	DATE WRITTEN	DATE OF SERVICE	FILL #	QTY DISPENSED (9)	DAYS SUPPLY

MM DD CCYY   MM DD CCYY

| PRODUCT / SERVICE I.D. | QUAL. (10) | DAW CODE | PRIOR AUTH # SUBMITTED | PA TYPE (11) | PRESCRIBER I.D. | QUAL. (12) |

DUR / PPS CODES (13)	BASIS COST (14)	PROVIDER I.D.	QUAL. (15)	DIAGNOSIS CODE	QUAL. (16)
A B C					

| OTHER PAYER DATE | OTHER PAYER I.D. | QUAL. (17) | OTHER PAYER REJECT CODES | USUAL & CUST. CHARGE |

MM DD CCYY

1

	INGREDIENT COST SUBMITTED
	DISPENSING FEE SUBMITTED
	INCENTIVE AMOUNT SUBMITTED
	OTHER AMOUNT SUBMITTED
	SALES TAX SUBMITTED
	GROSS AMOUNT DUE SUBMITTED
	PATIENT PAID AMOUNT
	OTHER PAYER AMOUNT PAID
	NET AMOUNT DUE

2

PRESCRIPTION / SERV. REF. #	QUAL. (8)	DATE WRITTEN	DATE OF SERVICE	FILL #	QTY DISPENSED (9)	DAYS SUPPLY

MM DD CCYY   MM DD CCYY

| PRODUCT / SERVICE I.D. | QUAL. (10) | DAW CODE | PRIOR AUTH # SUBMITTED | PA TYPE (11) | PRESCRIBER I.D. | QUAL. (12) |

DUR / PPS CODES (13)	BASIS COST (14)	PROVIDER I.D.	QUAL. (15)	DIAGNOSIS CODE	QUAL. (16)
A B C					

| OTHER PAYER DATE | OTHER PAYER I.D. | QUAL. (17) | OTHER PAYER REJECT CODES | USUAL & CUST. CHARGE |

MM DD CCYY

2

	INGREDIENT COST SUBMITTED
	DISPENSING FEE SUBMITTED
	INCENTIVE AMOUNT SUBMITTED
	OTHER AMOUNT SUBMITTED
	SALES TAX SUBMITTED
	GROSS AMOUNT DUE SUBMITTED
	PATIENT PAID AMOUNT
	OTHER PAYER AMOUNT PAID
	NET AMOUNT DUE

IMPORTANT: I certify that the patient information entered on the front side of this form is correct, that the patient named is eligible for the benefits and that I have received the medication described. If this claim is for a workers compensation injury, the appropriate section on the front side has been completed. I hereby assign the provider pharmacy any payment due pursuant to this transaction and authorize payment directly to the provider pharmacy. I also authorize release of all information pertainng to this claim to the plan administrator, underwriter, sponsor, policyholder and the employer.

PLEASE SIGN CERTIFICATION ON FRONT SIDE FOR PRESCRIPTION(S) RECEIVED

INSTRUCTIONS
1. Fill in all applicable areas on the front of this form.
2. Enter COMPOUND RX in the Product Service ID area(s) and list each ingredient, name, NDC, quantity, and cost in the area below.
   Please use a separate claim form for each compound prescription.
3. Worker's Comp. Information is conditional. It should be completed only for a Workers Comp. Claim.
4. Report diagnosis code and qualifier related to prescription (limit 1 per prescription).
5. Limit 1 set of DUR/PPS codes per claim.

DEFINITIONS / VALUES

1. OTHER COVERAGE CODE

0 = Not Specified	1 = No other coverage identified	2 = Other coverage exists – payment collected
3 = Other coverage exists – this claim not covered	4 = Other coverage exists – payment not collected	5 = Managed care plan denial
6 = Other coverage denied – not a participating provider	7 = Other coverage exists – not in effect at time of service	8 = Claim is billing for a co-pay

2. PERSON CODE: Code assigned to a specific person within a family.

3. PATIENT GENDER CODE

0 = Not Specified	1 = Male	2 = Female

4. PATIENT RELATIONSHIP CODE

0 = Not Specified	1 = Cardholder	2 = Spouse
3 = Child	4 = Other	

5. SERVICE PROVIDER ID QUALIFIER

Blank = Not Specified	01 = National Proider Identifier (NPI)	02 = Blue Cross
03 = Blue Shield	04 = Medicare	05 = Medicaid
06 = UPIN	07 = NCPDP Provider ID	08 = State License
09 = Champus	10 = Health Industry Number (HIN)	11 = Federal Tax ID
12 = Drug Enforcement Administration (DEA)	13 = State Issued	14 = Plan Specific
99 = Other		

6. CARRIER ID: Carrier code assigned in Worker's Compensation Program.

7. CLAIM/REFERENCE ID: Identifies the claim number assigned by Worker's Compensation Program.

8. PRESCRIPTION/SERVICE REFERENCE # QUALIFIER

Blank = Not Specified	1 = Rx billing	2 = Service billing

9. QUANTITY DISPENSED: Quantity dispensed expressed in metric decimal units (shaded areas for decimal values).

10. PRODUCT/SERVICE ID QUALIFIER: Code qualifying the value in Product/Service ID (407-07)

Blank = Not Specified	00 = Not Specified	01 = Universal Product Code (UPC)
02 = Health Related Item (HRI)	03 = National Drug Code (NDC)	04 = Universal Product Number (UPN)
05 = Department of Defense (DOD)	06 = Drug Use Review/Professional Pharm, Service (DUR/PPS)	07 = Common Procedure Terminology (CPT4)
08 = Common Procedure Terminology (CPT5)	09 = HCFA Common Procedural Coding System (HCPCS)	10 = Pharmacy Practice Activity Classification (PPAC)
11 = National Pharmaceutical Product Interface Code (NAPPI)	12 = International Article Numbering System (EAN)	13 = Drug Identification Number (DIN)
99 = Other		

11. PRIOR AUTHORIZATION TYPE CODE

0 = Not Specified	1 = Prior authorization	2 = Medical Certification
3 = EPSDT (Early Periodic Screening Diagnosis Treatment)	4 = Exemption from copay	5 = Exemption from Rx limits
6 = Family Planning Indicator	7 = Aid to Families with Dependent Children (AFDC)	8 = Payer Defined Exemption

12. PRESCRIBER ID QUALIFIER: Use service provider ID values.

13. DUR/PROFESSIONAL SERVICE CODES: Reason for Service, Professional Service Code, and Result of Service Codes. For values refer to current NCPDP data dictionary.

A = Reason for Service	B = Professional Service Code	C = Result of Service

14. BASIS OF COST DETERMINATION

Blank = Not Specified	00 = Not Specified	01 = AWP (Average Wholesale Price)
02 = Local Wholesaler	03 = Direct	04 = EAC (Estimated Acquisition Cost)
05 = Acquisition	06 = MAC (Maximum Allowable Cost)	07 = Usual & Customary
09 = Other		

15. PROVIDER ID QUALIFIER

Blank = Not Specified	01 = Drug Enforcement Administrator (DEA)	02 = State License
03 = Social Security Number (SSN)	04 = Name	05 = National Provider Identifier (NPI)
06 = Health Industry Number (HIN)	07 = State Issued	99 = Other

16. DIAGNOSIS CODE QUALIFIER

Blank = Not Specified	00 = Not Specified	01 = International Classification of Diseases (ICD9)
02 = International Classification of Diseases (ICD10)	03 = National Criteria Care Institute (NDCC)	04 = Systemized Nomenclature of Human and Veterinary Medicine (SNOMED)
05 = Common Dental Term (CDT)	06 = Medi-Span Diagnosis Code	07 = American Psychiatric Association Diagnostic Statistical Manual of Mental Disorders (DSM IV)
99 = Other		

17. OTHER PAYER ID QUALIFIER

Blank = Not Specified	01 = National Payer ID	02 = Health Industry Number (HIN)
03 = Bank Information Number (BIN)	04 = National Association of Insurance Commissioners (NAIC)	09 = Coupon
99 = Other		

COMPOUND PRESCRIPTIONS - LIMIT 1 COMPOUND PRESCRIPTION PER CLAIM FORM.

Name	NDC	Quantity	Cost

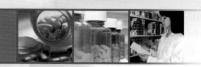

Patient and Physician Directory

PATIENT DIRECTORY

Thomas Aspen
D.O.B. 1/30/1940
1200 Waters Street
Tampa, Florida 33720
813-555-0132
Allergies: NKA
Smoker: No
INS: Walgreen13

Robin Copper
D.O.B. 12/10/1960
2145 Right Avenue
Test, Wyoming 82311
688-555-0154
Allergies: ASA, eggs
Smoker: Yes
INS: EXPRESSRX65

Traci Farmer
D.O.B. 06/20/1969
771 River Run Road
Spring Water, Tennessee 37328
618-555-0198
Allergies: PCN
Smoker: No
INS: AETNA51

Mike Fortuna
D.O. B. 09/10/1980
8080 Tall Oaks Road
Etowah, Tennessee 37371
612-555-0101
Allergies: NKA
Smoker: No
INS: Scrip-Card40

Bonnie Harris
D.O.B. 09/20/1985
6610 Woodlawn Street
St. Petersburg, Florida 33770
727-555-0173
Allergies: Latex
Smoker: No
INS: Selectscrip67t

Roger Horton
D.O.B. 08/16/1995
7721 Corbet Avenue
St. Petersburg, Florida 33710
727-555-0164
Allergies: TCN
Smoker: No
INS: Walgreen13

Wanda James
D.O.B. 04/15/1980
4010 Coastal Way
St. Petersburg, Florida 33770
727-555-0190
Allergies: NKA
Smoker: No
INS: Wellpoint55

William Johnson
D.O.B. 03/20/1945
4602 Coral Beach Drive
Clearwater, Florida 337716
727-555-0131
Allergies: APAP
Smoker: Yes
INS: Walgreen13

Tommy Klein
D.O.B. 02/10/1956
652 Bayway Drive
St. Petersburg, Florida 33715
727-555-0112
Allergies: Benzodiazepines
Smoker: Yes
INS: RXNET, Inc78

Ted Kline
D.O.B. 05/18/1943
9090 College Lane
Grandview, Alabama 32716
606-555-0121
Allergies: NKA
Smoker: No
INS: Walgreen13

George Roberts
D.O.B. 11/16/1955
613 Wilkerson Road
Spring Water, Tennessee 37328
618-555-0133
Allergies: ASA, wheat
Smoker: No
INS: MEDIMPACT5172

Lisa Rough
D.O.B. 06/10/1950
1316 Runner Way
Ocala, Florida 37370
612-555-0166
Allergies: NKA
Smoker: Yes
INS: Walgreen13

Kim Sands
D.O.B. 05/25/2001
4540 Kindle Lane
Hollywood, Florida 33895
804-555-0177
Allergies: Sulfa drugs
Smoker: No
INS: Med-Impact72

Greg Smith
D.O.B. 07/18/1990
845 North Iris Avenue
St. Petersburg, Florida 33701

727-555-0188
Allergies: NKA
Smoker: No
INS: AdvanceParadgm11

Mary Solvin
D.O.B. 07/20/1980
5828 49th Street
St. Petersburg, Florida 33710
727-555-0199
Allergies: Iodine
Smoker: Yes
INS: GHEA-PAIDRX82

Tammy Speed
D.O.B. 07/10/1995
1813 History Circle
Grandview, Alabama 32716
606-555-0102
Allergies: Codeine
Smoker: No
INS: Walgreen13

Bill Stevens
D.O.B. 05/10/1935
2610 Justin Street
Test, Wyoming 82000
688-555-0103
Allergies: Quinolones
Smoker: No
INS: MD-UNTDHLTH12

Ken Summer
D.O.B. 05/18/1970
765 Watson Road
Tarpon Springs, Florida 33720
727-555-0130
Allergies: Peanuts
Smoker: No
INS: MD-UNICARE19

Mary Taylor
D.O.B. 12/01/1989
9012 Intercoastal Way
St. Petersburg, Florida 33711
688-555-0104
Allergies: Sulfonamides, latex
Smoker: Yes
INS: Script-Card40

Bonnie Thompson
D.O.B. 10/13/1951
3015 Water Canal Street
Tarpon Springs, Florida 33720
727-555-0140
Allergies: Nitrates
Smoker: No
INS: Walgreen13

Chester Thompson
D.O.B. 12/01/1920
5858 Brookstone Road
St. Petersburg, Florida 33712
727-555-0105
Allergies: PCN
Smoker: No
INS: MD-CAREPLUS28

Sam Turner
D.O.B. 04/20/1970
9902 Reader Road
St. Petersburg, Florida 33706
688-555-0150
Allergies: Peanuts
Smoker: No
INS: MEDIMPACT5172

Susan Turner
D.O.B. 03/30/1970
8855 Corvette Avenue, Apt 10
St. Petersburg, Florida 33716
688-555-0134
Allergies: Eggs
Smoker: No
INS: Walgreen13

Karla Watts
D.O.B. 07/10/1999
192 Aspen Trail
Hollywood, Florida 33895
804-555-0106
Allergies: NKA
Smoker: No
INS: SCRIPT-CARD40

Grace Wilson
D.O.B. 03/24/1940
520 Grayson Road
St. Petersburg, Florida 33710

727-555-0160
Allergies: NKA
Smoker: Yes
INS: TRICARE-EXPRESS66

Jason Wilson
D.O.B. 07/16/1955
805 West Sumter Avenue
St. Petersburg, Florida 33714
727-555-0107
Allergies: NKA
Smoker: No
INS: MEDIMPACT5172

Joe Wilson
D.O.B. 09/15/1960
4050 Technology Way
Grandview, Florida 32715
727-555-0170
Allergies: Erythromycin
Smoker: Yes
INS: MD-UNTDHLTH12

Arnold Winston
D.O.B. 04/10/1930
1020 Turner Street
St. Petersburg, Florida 33712
688-555-0143
Allergies: PCN, latex
Smoker: Yes
INS: FED-BLXPCS91

Rose Winter
D.O.B. 02/12/1948
1120 Lakewood Road
Tampa, Florida 33710
727-555-0108
Allergies: Iodine
Smoker: Yes
INS: MD-CAREPLUS28

Selina Wright
D.O.B. 08/25/1945
2625 Throughbred Street
Spring Waters, Tennessee 37328
618-555-0180
Allergies: Eggs
Smoker: No
INS: Walgreen13

Name of Physician or Clinic
Address
Office Phone Number
Fax Number

Patient Information:

Name: _____ M / F
        Last   First   Middle   (Circle One)

Mailing Address: _____
                Address   City   State   Zip

Home Phone: _____ Work Phone: _____

Date of Birth: _____ SS#: _____

Marital Status: Single / Married / Widowed / Divorced (please circle one)

Insurance Information:

Relationship of Patient to Insured: _____Self _____Spouse _____Child _____Other (explain): _____

Primary Insurance: _____

Policy Holder: _____ Phone:_____

Mailing Address: _____
                Address   City   State   Zip

Date of Birth of Policy Holder: _____ SS# of Policy Holder: _____

Policy Holders Employer: _____ Phone: (_____)_____

. . . .

Secondary Insurance: _____

Secondary Policy Holder: _____ Phone:_____

Mailing Address: _____
                Address   City   State   Zip

Date of Birth of Policy Holder: _____ SS# of Policy Holder: _____

Policy Holders Employer: _____ Phone: (_____)_____

Emergency Contact: _____ Relation: _____

Phone Number of Contact: _____

I understand and agree that (regardless of my insurance status), I am responsible for the balance of my account. I have read the information on this sheet and have completed the above answers. I certify that this information is true and correct to the best of my knowledge.

Signature: _____ Date: _____

PHYSICIAN DIRECTORY

William Astor, M.D.
Cardiologist
1418 West River Road
Spring Waters, Tennessee 37328
618-555-0155
FAX 618-555-0111

Brian Bonea, M.D.
Rheumatologist
123 Test Street
Test, Wyoming 82000
688-555-0145
FAX 688-555-0114

James Campbell, M.D.
Pediatrician
9080 Turner Street
Hollywood, Florida 33896
804-555-0122
FAX 804-555-0139

Mac U. Feelgoud, M.D.
General Surgery
1234 West Lerner Street
St. Petersburg, Florida 33716
727-555-0189
FAX 727-555-0138

Jason Jones, M.D.
Internal Medicine Specialist
469 Medical Circle, Suite B
Ocala, Florida 37370
612-555-0137
FAX 612-555-0115

Russell Livingston, D.O.
General Medicine
987 Circle Back Way
Tarpon Springs, Florida 33720
727-555-0146
FAX 727-555-0136

Roger Lowell, M.D.
Orthopedic Surgeon
8020 University Circle

Grandview, Alabama 32716
606-555-0109
FAX 606-555-0116

Kathy O'Conner, D.O.
Internal Medicine Specialist
2345 Miller Road Way
St. Petersburg, Florida 33716
727-555-0144
FAX 727-555-0119

Scott Smith, M.D.
Internal Medicine Specialist
1234 West Lerner Street
St. Petersburg, Florida 33716
727-555-0123
FAX 727-555-0129

Markus Welby, M.D.
General Practitioner
1234 West Lerner Street
St. Petersburg, Florida 33716
688-555-0110
FAX 688-555-0117

Jane Wester, M.D.
Gerontology
8080 West Lane, Suite A
St. Petersburg, Florida 33716
727-555-0113
FAX 727-555-0128

Thomas Westfield, M.D.
Gastroenterologist
1234 Halfwater Avenue
St. Petersburg, Florida 33716
727-555-0167
FAX 727-555-0118

Joyce White, D.O.
Ophthalmologist
6789 Lester Avenue, Suite A
Tampa, Florida 33711
813-555-0176
FAX 813-584-4478

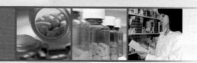

Medication Administration Forms

Examples of a variety of medication administration forms, Physician's Orders, and treatment orders.

DATE 05/16/XX	Resident Name: ROUTINE, ORDERS	**PHYSICIAN'S ORDER**	ORIGINAL

ORDERS	FREQ.
D/C _____ Order# 00016 01) (_)-PPD MANTOUX: TEST ID NOW AND IF NEGATIVE REPEAT IN 7 DAYS AND ANNUALLY. MONTH:_____ (S-CTPPD) ICD9 Diagnosis	
D/C _____ Order# 00017 02) (_)-PNEUMOVAX: INJECT 0.5ML IM OR SC X1 DOSE IF NOT RECEIVED IN LAST 5 YEARS ICD9 Diagnosis	
D/C _____ Order# 00018 03) (_)-TETANUS TOXOID ADSORBED: INJECT 0.5ML IM X1 DOSE IF NOT GIVEN IN LAST 10 YEARS ICD9 Diagnosis	
ICD9 Diagnosis	
ICD9 Diagnosis	
ICD9 Diagnosis	
ICD9 Diagnosis	

DOCTOR

RESIDENT

DATE
ROOM #
ALLERGIES

OTHER ODERS

ACTIVITIES AND MOBILITY:
(_)-YES. (_)-NO.............. PHYSICAL
&.SOCIAL.ACTIVITIES.AS TOLERATED
(_)-WITH.ASSIST.OR.DEVICE (_)-BED.TO.CHAIR.
(_)-UP.IN.CHAIR-FREQUENCY_____ (S-CTACTIV)

(_)-YES.(_)-NO........... LEAVE OF ABSENCE AS
NEEDED (S-CTLOA)

CONSULTATIONS & THERAPIES:
PODIATRY, DENTAL, OPHTHALMIC.. CONSULTATIONS
AS.NEEDED OTHER:_____
(S-CTCONSULT)

UNIVERSAL ORDERS:
DR ORDERS, PATIENT CARE PLAN, ACTIVITIES &
DISCHARGE REVIEWED & APPROVED

NURSE MAY CHECK FOR CONSTIPATION AND PROVIDE
DIGITAL STIMULATION AS NEEDED

MAY CHANGE BETWEEN ORAL SOLIDS / LIQUIDS / OPEN
CAPSULES OR CRUSH TABS UNLESS CONTRAINDICATED
OR GIVE VIA ENTERAL TUBE IF TUBE IN PLACE

DIETARY CONSISTENCY MAY BE CHANGED AS CONDITION
WARRANTS

MAY BATHE IN CENTURY TUB, SHOWER OR WHIRLPOOL

WEIGHT: RECORD AT LEAST EACH MONTH & REPORT 5%
DIFFERENCE TO PHYSICIAN

URINARY CATHETER ORDERS:
MAY STRAIGHT CATH TO OBTAIN U/A AS NEEDED
(S-CTCATH)

ROUTINE ORDERS:

PRESCRIBER SIGNATURE _____ DATE _____

REVIEWED BY _____ DATE _____ NOTED BY _____ DATE _____

TOTAL RX: 0	TOTAL ROUTINES: 0	TOTAL PRN: 0
	TOTAL RTN TRMT: 0	TOTAL PRN TRMT: 0

*
*

REVIEW OF ENTIRE DRUG REGIMEN AND COMPREHENSIVE
RESIDENT CARE PLAN IS COMPLETED.

ANY IRREGULARITIES ARE DOCUMENTED IN THE
PHARMACIST'S MONTHLY REPORTS.

X
PHARMACY   DATE

☐ NO IRREGULARITIES NOTED
☐ INSIGNIFICANT IRREGULARITIES NOTED
☐ SIGNIFICANT IRREGULARITIES NOTED

☐ SEND * MEDS ONLY   ☐ SEND NO MEDS   ☐ SEND ALL MEDS

FIN PLAN-   SEX- M   DOB-
  NH RES#-   RES CODE- 96027

ROUTINE, ORDERS

DATE	Resident ENTERAL, ORDERS	**PHYSICIAN'S ORDER**	
05/28/XX	Name:		ORIGINAL

ORDERS	FREQ.	OTHER ODERS
D/C _____ Order# 00001 1)-ENTERAL FEEDING:_____ AT _____ML/HR. TOTAL CALORIES:_____(CTEN1) ICD9 Diagnosis		****ENTERAL ORDERS****: . .
D/C _____ Order# 00002 2)-CHECK TUBE PLACEMENT EVERY 4 HOURS AND WITH ADDITIVES & PO MDS VIA ENTERAL TUBE WHILE IN PLACE (CTEN2) ICD9 Diagnosis		. .
D/C _____ Order# 00003 3)-ENTERAL FLUSH WITH _____ML OF _____EVERY _____HOURS (CTEN3) ICD9 Diagnosis		. .
D/C _____ Order# 00004 4)-TUBE TYPE:_____ & CHANGE:_____ (CTEN4) ICD9 Diagnosis		. .
D/C _____ Order# 00005 5)-CHANGE SET DAILY & AS NEEDED (CTEN5) ICD9 Diagnosis		. .
D/C _____ Order# 00006 6)-ELEVATE HEAD OF BED AT 30 DEGREES AT ALL TIMES (CTEN6) ICD9 Diagnosis		. .
D/C _____ Order# 00007 7)-ORAL AND NASAL CARE EVERY SHIFT (CTEN7) ICD9 Diagnosis		. .
   ICD9 Diagnosis		. .

DIAGNOSIS

DOCTOR   DATE
                         ROOM #
RESIDENT   ALLERGIES

.
.
.
.
.
.

PRESCRIBER SIGNATURE _____ DATE _____

REVIEWED BY _____ DATE _____ NOTED BY _____ DATE _____

TOTAL RX: 0	TOTAL ROUTINES: 0	TOTAL PRN: 0	REVIEW OF ENTIRE DRUG REGIMEN AND COMPREHENSIVE RESIDENT CARE PLAN IS COMPLETED.	☐ NO IRREGULARITIES NOTED
	TOTAL RTN TRMT: 0	TOTAL PRN TRMT: 0		☐ INSIGNIFICANT IRREGULARITIES NOTED
*			ANY IRREGULARITIES ARE DOCUMENTED IN THE PHARMACIST'S MONTHLY REPORTS.	☐ SIGNIFICANT IRREGULARITIES NOTED
*			X_____	
			PHARMACY	DATE

☐ SEND * MEDS ONLY   ☐ SEND NO MEDS   ☐ SEND ALL MEDS

FIN PLAN-   SEX- M   DOB-
  NH RES#-   RES CODE- 80796

ENTERAL, ORDERS

| DATE 06/26/XX | Resident CATHETER, ORDERS Name: | **PHYSICIAN'S ORDER** | ORIGINAL |

ORDERS	FREQ.	OTHER ODERS
D/C _____ Order# 00001 1)-IRRIGATE CATHETER WITH ...ML OF .... AS NEEDED FOR LEAKAGE OR BLOCKAGE (CTCA1) ICD9 Diagnosis		**CATHETER ORDERS**: . . .
D/C _____ Order# 00002 2)-CHANGE CATHETER #..FR/..CC (+/- 1 SIZE) AS NEEDED FOR LEAKAGE OR BLOCKAGE (CTCA2) ICD9 Diagnosis		. .
D/C _____ Order# 00003 3)-REASON FOR CATHETER:............. (CTCA3) ICD9 Diagnosis		. .
D/C _____ Order# 00004 4)-CHANGE DRAINAGE BAG WEEKLY ON SUNDAY (CTCA4) ICD9 Diagnosis		.
ICD9 Diagnosis		.
ICD9 Diagnosis		.
ICD9 Diagnosis		.

DIAGNOSIS

DOCTOR   DATE

                             ROOM #

RESIDENT   ALLERGIES

PRESCRIBER SIGNATURE _____ DATE _____

REVIEWED BY _____ DATE _____ NOTED BY _____ DATE _____

TOTAL RX: 0	TOTAL ROUTINES: 0	TOTAL PRN: 0	REVIEW OF ENTIRE DRUG REGIMEN AND COMPREHENSIVE RESIDENT CARE PLAN IS COMPLETED.	☐ NO IRREGULARITIES NOTED
	TOTAL RTN TRMT: 0	TOTAL PRN TRMT: 0		☐ INSIGNIFICANT IRREGULARITIES NOTED
*			ANY IRREGULARITIES ARE DOCUMENTED IN THE PHARMACIST'S MONTHLY REPORTS.	☐ SIGNIFICANT IRREGULARITIES NOTED
*			X _____	
			PHARMACY	DATE

☐ SEND * MEDS ONLY   ☐ SEND NO MEDS   ☐ SEND ALL MEDS

FIN PLAN-   SEX- M   DOB-
  NH RES#-   RES CODE- 80797

CATHETER, ORDERS

See Reverse Side For Verifying Signatures

Routine Orders
RESIDENT "CHEEKS" MEDS

04/01/20XX

| | FREQUENCY: | 1 | 2 | 3 | 4 | 5 | 6 | 7 | 8 | 9 | 10 | 11 | 12 | 13 | 14 | 15 | 16 | 17 | 18 | 19 | 20 | 21 | 22 | 23 | 24 | 25 | 26 | 27 | 28 | 29 | 30 | 31 |

01/25/20XX RX 309632
ARTIFICIAL TEARS 15CC DROPS

INSTILL 2 DROPS IN BOTH EYES TWO TIMES A DAY

FREQUENCY:
09:00
18:00

01/25/20XX RX 309633
FERROUS SULFATE 325MG TAB   325MG

1 TABLET BY MOUTH TWICE DAILY WITH FOOD

FREQUENCY:
10:00
16:00

SE: Stomach Pain/cramps; Constipation; Nausea; Vomiting; Diar

01/25/20XX RX 309634
FUROSEMIDE 40MG TABLET   40MG
-I.E. LASIX 40MG TABLET   40MG
1 TABLET BY MOUTH TWICE DAILY

FREQUENCY:
08:00
18:00

SE: Orthostatic Hypotension; Hyponatremia; Hypokalemia

01/25/20XX RX 309635
K-DUR 20MEQ TABLET SA   20MEQ

1 TABLET BY MOUTH TWICE DAILY

FREQUENCY:
09:00
17:00

SE: Vomiting; Gas; Diarrhea; Stomach Pain; Discomfort; Hyperk

01/25/20XX RX 309636
PLAVIX 75MG TABLET   75MG

ONE TABLET BY MOUTH ONCE DAILY

FREQUENCY:
07:30

SE: Purpura; Upper Respiratory Infection; Pain; Chest Pain

04/23/20XX
DO -NOT- RESUSCITATE

FREQUENCY:

LOA WITH SUPERVISION & MEDS

PHYSICIAN: MADDEN, WILLIAM   937-233-2888
ALT. PHYS: DR. R. SMITH   937-223-2901
                                  DOB- 05/06/1933
                                  ADM- 12-AB467
                                  ACC- 017001
                                  RM#   212A

PARKINSON'S; HTN; HX DEPRESSION W/ANXIETY; DELUSIONAL DISORDER;
CHF; IRON DEFICIENCY ANEMIA; HYPOKALEMIA; CONSTIPATION; EDEMA;

WOOL; MOHAIR

SAMPLE FACILITY - STATION 1   CPG PHARMACY

ADAMS, MARY

Page 1

Nurse's Medication Notes

Instructions:

A. SUGGEST REFUSED / WITHHELD MEDICATION EXPLAINED IN NURSES MEDICATION NOTES.

B. WHEN PRN MEDICATIONS ARE GIVEN, EXPLAIN IN NURSES MEDICATION NOTES.

Indicate Site With Appropriate Number:

1. BUTTOCKS (GLUTEUS) LEFT
2. BUTTOCKS (GLUTEUS) RIGHT
3. ARM (DELTOID) LEFT
4. ARM (DELTOID) RIGHT
5. THIGH (QUADRICEPS) LEFT
6. THIGH (QUADRICEPS) RIGHT
7. ABDOMEN LEFT
8. ABDOMEN RIGHT
9. UPPER BACK LEFT
10. UPPER BACK RIGHT
11. UPPER CHEST LEFT
12. UPPER CHEST RIGHT

RESULT CODES

B = BM RESULTED
E = EFFECTIVE
I = INEFFECTIVE
N = SEE NURSES NOTES
R = WITH RELIEF
S = SLEEP RESULTED

Date	Time	Init.	Drug - Strength - Dose	Site	Reason	Result	Date	Time	Obser. Init.

Signature & Title	Initials	Signature & Title	Initials

See Reverse Side For Verifying Signatures

PRN Orders
RESIDENT "CHEEKS" MEDS

04/01/20XX

01/25/20XX RX 309628
ACETAMINOPHEN 325MG TABLET   325MG
-I.E. TYLENOL 325MG   325MG
1 TABLET EVERY 4hrs AS NEEDED ELEV. TEMP
>101F

FREQUENCY: 15 16 17 18 19 20 21 22 23 24 25 26 27 28 29 30 1 2 3 4 5 6 7 8 9 10 11 12 13 14 | 31

SE: Anemia; Thrombocytopenia; Agranulocytosis; Hepatitis;

01/25/20XX RX 309629
BISACODYL 10MG SUPPOSITORY

1 RECTALLY PRN CONSTIPATION IF MOM NOT
EFFECTIVE AFTER 24HRS

FREQUENCY: 15 16 17 18 19 20 21 22 23 24 25 26 27 28 29 30 1 2 3 4 5 6 7 8 9 10 11 12 13 14 | 31

SE: Perianal Irritation; Nausea; Belching; Diarrhea; Cramps;

01/25/20XX RX 309630
MILK OF MAGNESIA - PHILLIPS

30CC BY MOUTH DAILY AS NEEDED IF NO B.M.
AFTER 2 DAYS

FREQUENCY: 15 16 17 18 19 20 21 22 23 24 25 26 27 28 29 30 1 2 3 4 5 6 7 8 9 10 11 12 13 14 | 31

SE: Increased Thirst; Gas; Diarrhea; Stomach Cramps;

FREQUENCY: 1 2 3 4 5 6 7 8 9 10 11 12 13 14 15 16 17 18 19 20 21 22 23 24 25 26 27 28 29 30 31

FREQUENCY: 1 2 3 4 5 6 7 8 9 10 11 12 13 14 15 16 17 18 19 20 21 22 23 24 25 26 27 28 29 30 31

FREQUENCY: 1 2 3 4 5 6 7 8 9 10 11 12 13 14 15 16 17 18 19 20 21 22 23 24 25 26 27 28 29 30 31

FREQUENCY: 1 2 3 4 5 6 7 8 9 10 11 12 13 14 15 16 17 18 19 20 21 22 23 24 25 26 27 28 29 30 31

Page 1

PHYSICIAN: MADDEN, WILLIAM   937-233-2888   PARKINSON'S; HTN; HX DEPRESSION W/ANXIETY; DELUSIONAL DISORDER;
ALT. PHYS: DR. R. SMITH   937-223-2901   CHF; IRON DEFICIENCY ANEMIA; HYPOKALEMIA; CONSTIPATION; EDEMA;
                                  DOB- 05/06/1933
                                  ADM- 12-AB467   WOOL; MOHAIR
                                  ACC- 017001
                                  RM# 212A   SAMPLE FACILITY - STATION 1   CPG PHARMACY

ADAMS, MARY

COMMENTS

Instructions:

A. WHEN PRNS ARE GIVEN, EXPLAIN IN NURSES NOTES.

B. SUGGEST REFUSED / WITHHELD MEDICATION EXPLAINED IN NURSES MEDICATION NOTES.

Date	Time	Initial	Comments

Date	Time	Initial	Comments

INITIALS	FULL SIGNATURE	TITLE	INITIALS	FULL SIGNATURE	TITLE

See Reverse Side For Verifying Signatures

Treatment Orders
RESIDENT "CHEEKS" MEDS

04/01/20XX

01/25/20XX RX 310243
ARISTOCORT A 0.1% CREAM   0.1%

APPLY TO RASH ON FOREHEAD AS NEEDED -
ITCHING

FREQUENCY 15 16 17 18 19 20 21 22 23 24 25 26 27 28 29 30 1 2 3 4 5 6 7 8 9 10 11 12 13 14
P
R
N

SE: Purpura; Telangiectasia; Furunculosis; Pyoderma; Skin Inf

01/25/20XX
APPLY VASELINE LOTION TO ELBOWS AND
KNEES TWICE DAILY

FREQUENCY 15 16 17 18 19 20 21 22 23 24 25 26 27 28 29 30 1 2 3 4 5 6 7 8 9 10 11 12 13 14
7AM
3PM

01/27/20XX
APPLY TED HOSE (THIGH HIGH) EVERY MORNING
AND REMOVE AT BEDTIME

FREQUENCY 15 16 17 18 19 20 21 22 23 24 25 26 27 28 29 30 1 2 3 4 5 6 7 8 9 10 11 12 13 14
ON
OFF

FREQUENCY:

FREQUENCY:

FREQUENCY:

FREQUENCY:

FREQUENCY:

Page 1

PHYSICIAN: MADDEN, WILLIAM   937-233-2888
ALT. PHYS: DR. R. SMITH   937-223-2901
                                 DOB- 05/06/1933
                                 ADM- 12-AB467
                                 ACC- 017001
                                 RM# 212A

ADAMS, MARY

PARKINSON'S; HTN; HX DEPRESSION W/ANXIETY; DELUSIONAL DISORDER;
CHF; IRON DEFICIENCY ANEMIA; HYPOKALEMIA; CONSTIPATION; EDEMA;

WOOL; MOHAIR

SAMPLE FACILITY - STATION 1   CPG PHARMACY

COMMENTS

Instructions:

A. WHEN PRNS ARE GIVEN, EXPLAIN IN NURSES NOTES.

B. SUGGEST REFUSED / WITHHELD MEDICATION
   EXPLAINED IN NURSES MEDICATION NOTES.

Date	Time	Initial	Comments

Date	Time	Initial	Comments

INITIALS	FULL SIGNATURE	TITLE	INITIALS	FULL SIGNATURE	TITLE

INITIALS	FULL SIGNATURE	TITLE	INITIALS	FULL SIGNATURE	TITLE

ADMINISTRATION RECORD

DATE	
05/28/XX	

Resident ENTERAL, ORDERS
Name:

MAY03

ORDERS | **FREQ.** | 1 2 3 4 5 6 7 8 9 10 11 12 13 14 15 16 17 18 19 20 21 22 23 24 25 26 27 28 29 30 31

D/C _____ Order# 00001 _____ AT _____ ML/HR.
1)-ENTERAL FEEDING: _____
TOTAL CALORIES: _____ (CTEN1)

D/C _____ Order# 00002
2)-CHECK TUBE PLACEMENT EVERY 4 HOURS AND WITH
ADDITIVES & PO MDS VIA ENTERAL TUBE WHILE IN
PLACE (CTEN2)

D/C _____ Order# 00003 _____ EVERY
3)-ENTERAL FLUSH WITH _____ ML OF _____
_____ HOURS (CTEN3)

D/C _____ Order# 00004 _____ (CTEN4)
4)-TUBE TYPE: _____ & CHANGE: _____

D/C _____ Order# 00005
5)-CHANGE SET DAILY & AS NEEDED (CTEN5)

D/C _____ Order# 00006
6)-ELEVATE HEAD OF BED AT 30 DEGREES AT ALL
TIMES (CTEN6)

D/C _____ Order# 00007
7)-ORAL AND NASAL CARE EVERY SHIFT (CTEN7)

DIAGNOSIS

DOCTOR

DATE

ROOM #

RESIDENT

ALLERGIES

REVIEW OF ENTIRE DRUG REGIMEN
AND COMPREHENSIVE RESIDENT
CARE PLAN IS COMPLETED.

ANY IRREGULARITIES ARE DOCUMENTED
IN THE PHARMACIST'S MONTHLY REPORTS.

☐ NO IRREGULARITIES NOTED
☐ INSIGNIFICANT IRREGULARITIES NOTED
☐ SIGNIFICANT IRREGULARITIES NOTED

X _____
PHARMACY

_____ _____
DATE

COMMENTS

Instructions:

A. WHEN PRNS ARE GIVEN, EXPLAIN IN NURSES NOTES.

B. SUGGEST REFUSED / WITHHELD MEDICATION EXPLAINED IN NURSES MEDICATION NOTES.

Date	Time	Initial	Comments

Date	Time	Initial	Comments

INITIALS	FULL SIGNATURE	TITLE	INITIALS	FULL SIGNATURE	TITLE

INITIALS	FULL SIGNATURE	TITLE	INITIALS	FULL SIGNATURE	TITLE

INDEX

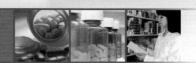

IMPORTANT! READ CAREFULLY: This End User License Agreement ("Agreement") sets forth the conditions by which Cengage Learning will make electronic access to the Cengage Learning-owned licensed content and associated media, software, documentation, printed materials, and electronic documentation contained in this package and/or made available to you via this product (the "Licensed Content"), available to you (the "End User"). BY CLICKING THE "I ACCEPT" BUTTON AND/OR OPENING THIS PACKAGE, YOU ACKNOWLEDGE THAT YOU HAVE READ ALL OF THE TERMS AND CONDITIONS, AND THAT YOU AGREE TO BE BOUND BY ITS TERMS, CONDITIONS,AND ALL APPLICABLE LAWS AND REGULATIONS GOVERNING THE USE OF THE LICENSED CONTENT.

1.0 SCOPE OF LICENSE

1.1   Licensed Content. The Licensed Content may contain portions of modifiable content ("Modifiable Content") and content which may not be modified or otherwise altered by the End User ("Non-Modifiable Content"). For purposes of this Agreement, Modifiable Content and Non-Modifiable Content may be collectively referred to herein as the "Licensed Content." All Licensed Content shall be considered Non-Modifiable Content, unless such Licensed Content is presented to the End User in a modifiable format and it is clearly indicated that modification of the Licensed Content is permitted.

1.2   Subject to the End User's compliance with the terms and conditions of this Agreement, Cengage Learning hereby grants the End User, a nontransferable, nonexclusive, limited right to access and view a single copy of the Licensed Content on a single personal computer system for noncommercial, internal, personal use only. The End User shall not (i) reproduce, copy, modify (except in the case of Modifiable Content), distribute, display, transfer, sublicense, prepare derivative work(s) based on, sell, exchange, barter or transfer, rent, lease, loan, resell, or in any other manner exploit the Licensed Content; (ii) remove, obscure, or alter any notice of Cengage Learning's intellectual property rights present on or in the Licensed Content, including, but not limited to, copyright, trademark, and/or patent notices; or (iii) disassemble, decompile, translate, reverse engineer, or otherwise reduce the Licensed Content.

2.0 TERMINATION

2.1   Cengage Learning may at any time (without prejudice to its other rights or remedies) immediately terminate this Agreement and/or suspend access to some or all of the Licensed Content, in the event that the End User does not comply with any of the terms and conditions of this Agreement. In the event of such termination by Cengage Learning, the End User shall immediately return any and all copies of the Licensed Content to Cengage Learning.

3.0 PROPRIETARY RIGHTS

3.1   The End User acknowledges that Cengage Learning owns all rights, title and interest, including, but not limited to all copyright rights therein, in and to the Licensed Content, and that the End User shall not take any action inconsistent with such ownership. The Licensed Content is protected by U.S., Canadian and other applicable copyright laws and by international treaties, including the Berne Convention and the Universal Copyright Convention. Nothing contained in this Agreement shall be construed as granting the End User any ownership rights in or to the Licensed Content.

3.2   Cengage Learning reserves the right at any time to withdraw from the Licensed Content any item or part of an item for which it no longer retains the right to publish, or which it has reasonable grounds to believe infringes copyright or is defamatory, unlawful, or otherwise objectionable.

4.0 PROTECTION AND SECURITY

4.1   The End User shall use its best efforts and take all reasonable steps to safeguard its copy of the Licensed Content to ensure that no unauthorized reproduction, publication, disclosure, modification, or distribution of the Licensed Content, in whole or in part, is made. To the extent that the End User becomes aware of any such unauthorized use of the Licensed Content, the End User shall immediately notify Cengage Learning. Notification of such violations may be made by sending an e-mail to infringement@cengage.com.

5.0 MISUSE OF THE LICENSED PRODUCT

5.1   In the event that the End User uses the Licensed Content in violation of this Agreement, Cengage Learning shall have the option of electing liquidated damages, which shall include all profits generated by the End User's use of the Licensed Content plus interest computed at the maximum rate permitted by law and all legal fees and other expenses incurred by Cengage Learning in enforcing its rights, plus penalties.

6.0 FEDERAL GOVERNMENT CLIENTS

6.1 Except as expressly authorized by Cengage Learning, Federal Government clients obtain only the rights specified in this Agreement and no other rights. The Government acknowledges that (i) all software and related documentation incorporated in the Licensed Content is existing commercial computer software within the meaning of FAR 27.405(b)(2); and (2) all other data delivered in whatever form, is limited rights data within the meaning of FAR 27.401. The restrictions in this section are acceptable as consistent with the Government's need for software and other data under this Agreement.

7.0 DISCLAIMER OF WARRANTIES AND LIABILITIES

7.1 Although Cengage Learning believes the Licensed Content to be reliable, Cengage Learning does not guarantee or warrant (i) any information or materials contained in or produced by the Licensed Content, (ii) the accuracy, completeness or reliability of the Licensed Content, or (iii) that the Licensed Content is free from errors or other material defects. THE LICENSED PRODUCT IS PROVIDED "AS IS," WITHOUT ANY WARRANTY OF ANY KIND AND CENGAGE LEARNING DISCLAIMS ANY AND ALL WARRANTIES, EXPRESSED OR IMPLIED, INCLUDING, WITHOUT LIMITATION, WARRANTIES OF MERCHANTABILITY OR FITNESS FOR A PARTICULAR PURPOSE. IN NO EVENT SHALL CENGAGE LEARNING BE LIABLE FOR: INDIRECT, SPECIAL, PUNITIVE OR CONSEQUENTIAL DAMAGES INCLUDING FOR LOST PROFITS, LOST DATA, OR OTHERWISE. IN NO EVENT SHALL CENGAGE LEARNING'S AGGREGATE LIABILITY HEREUNDER, WHETHER ARISING IN CONTRACT, TORT, STRICT LIABILITY OR OTHERWISE, EXCEED THE AMOUNT OF FEES PAID BY THE END USER HEREUNDER FOR THE LICENSE OF THE LICENSED CONTENT.

8.0 GENERAL

8.1 <u>Entire Agreement</u>. This Agreement shall constitute the entire Agreement between the Parties and supercedes all prior Agreements and understandings oral or written relating to the subject matter hereof.

8.2 <u>Enhancements/Modifications of Licensed Content</u>. From time to time, and in Cengage Learning's sole discretion, Cengage Learning may advise the End User of updates, upgrades, enhancements and/or improvements to the Licensed Content, and may permit the End User to access and use, subject to the terms and conditions of this Agreement, such modifications, upon payment of prices as may be established by Cengage Learning.

8.3 <u>No Export</u>. The End User shall use the Licensed Content solely in the United States and shall not transfer or export, directly or indirectly, the Licensed Content outside the United States.

8.4 <u>Severability</u>. If any provision of this Agreement is invalid, illegal, or unenforceable under any applicable statute or rule of law, the provision shall be deemed omitted to the extent that it is invalid, illegal, or unenforceable. In such a case, the remainder of the Agreement shall be construed in a manner as to give greatest effect to the original intention of the parties hereto.

8.5 <u>Waiver</u>. The waiver of any right or failure of either party to exercise in any respect any right provided in this Agreement in any instance shall not be deemed to be a waiver of such right in the future or a waiver of any other right under this Agreement.

8.6 <u>Choice of Law/Venue</u>. This Agreement shall be interpreted, construed, and governed by and in accordance with the laws of the State of New York, applicable to contracts executed and to be wholly preformed therein, without regard to its principles governing conflicts of law. Each party agrees that any proceeding arising out of or relating to this Agreement or the breach or threatened breach of this Agreement may be commenced and prosecuted in a court in the State and County of New York. Each party consents and submits to the nonexclusive personal jurisdiction of any court in the State and County of New York in respect of any such proceeding.

8.7 <u>Acknowledgment</u>. By opening this package and/or by accessing the Licensed Content on this Web site, THE END USER ACKNOWLEDGES THAT IT HAS READ THIS AGREEMENT, UNDERSTANDS IT, AND AGREES TO BE BOUND BY ITS TERMS AND CONDITIONS. IF YOU DO NOT ACCEPT THESE TERMS AND CONDITIONS, YOU MUST NOT ACCESS THE LICENSED CONTENT AND RETURN THE LICENSED PRODUCT TO CENGAGE LEARNING (WITHIN 30 CALENDAR DAYS OF THE END USER'S PURCHASE) WITH PROOF OF PAYMENT ACCEPTABLE TO CENGAGE LEARNING, FOR A CREDIT OR A REFUND. Should the End User have any questions/comments regarding this Agreement, please contact Cengage Learning at Delmar.help@cengage.com.